KU-680-959

CONTENTS

PREFACE TO SECOND EDITION

During the 6 years since the publication of the first edition, there has been a considerable increase in the world literature on speech and language disorders, and also a growing interest in the field of neuro-linguistics. It is not the authors' aim with this book to provide a comprehensive review but rather to present in simplified form the neurological aspects of speech. In this edition there is a re-arrangement of chapters and the book is now divided into two parts.

In Part 1, the brain, its functions and their derangements, and the various types of speech and language disorders are described.

Part 2 gives a concise account of brain disorders which can influence speech and language. Only those anatomical, physiological and pathological details required for the understanding of basic neurology have been included, and reference to larger text books will be needed for more comprehensive accounts of neurological disorders. However, we hope that this small volume will make this difficult subject more readily understandable for those concerned with the neurological aspects of communication.

Few books satisfy both student and specialist. The first edition, being based on our lectures to schools of speech therapy and on subsequent experience as examiners in neurology for the College of Speech Therapists and University of Newcastle upon Tyne, seemed to have filled a gap for student and practising speech therapists. As a basic text, the book has to be reasonably inexpensive and act as a guide to the more specialised works referred to in the bibliography.

We are grateful for the constructive criticism of the reviewers of the previous edition, and for helpful discussions with our neurologist and speech therapist colleagues. Many suggestions have been incorporated into this edition and chapters have been enlarged, e.g. memory and amnesia (Chapter 3), the part of laryngeal reflexes in the mechanism of stammering (Chapter 8) and dysphonia (Chapter 12). A chapter has been added on trauma in view of its importance as a cause of speech disorders.

We are grateful to the Librarian at the Nottingham General Hospital for checking the bibliography and also to the Departments of Medical Illustration at the Nottingham General and Charing Cross Hospitals for help with the diagrams.

We are also indebted once again to our secretaries for their help with the manuscript, to Mr. Brian Armitage for preparing the index and to the publishers for the production of this book.

PREFACE TO FIRST EDITION

There is a vast literature on the many disciplines with which speech is concerned, but this book is intended as a simple presentation of the neurological approach to its anatomy, physiology and pathology. Although based on courses of lectures given by the authors in three of the schools of speech therapy in Great Britain, it should prove helpful not only to speech therapists, both for their final examinations and for practice afterwards, but also to medical students and others in disciplines concerned with communication, e.g. paediatrics, psychiatry, psychology, phonetics and linguistics.

The neurological mechanisms of speech and its disorders are complex and because of our pragmatic simplification a selected bibliography is given.

It is a pleasure to acknowledge our indebtedness to our teachers and colleagues who are too numerous to mention individually. We are particularly grateful to Professor W. Ritchie Russell and the Clarendon Press for permission to quote from the book *Traumatic Aphasia*, and also to Dr. Macdonald Critchley and the late Lord Brain for their teaching and literature.

We also thank the authors and publishers who have given permission for the reproduction of the illustrations acknowledged in the text. We are grateful to Dr. Paul Millac for reading the proofs and making helpful suggestions, and to Mr. B. Armitage, Librarian at the Charing Cross Hospital Medical School for preparing the index.

Our thanks are due to Mrs. Vanessa Dussek and Mrs. Patricia Espir for their patience in typing and retyping the chapters, and to the Department of Medical Illustration of Charing Cross Hospital for help with diagrams.

PART 1

CHAPTER 1

INTRODUCTION

Speech is unique to man. It can be defined as a system of communication in which thoughts are expressed and understood by using acoustic symbols. They are produced by the vibration of the vocal cords in the larynx (phonation), caused by the flow of air (respiration) and given final form by movements of the lips, tongue and palate (articulation).

Speech refers to verbal symbols, but language includes the non-verbal aspects of communication, for example—gesticulation, gesture and pantomine, each of which is different. Gesticulation is the associated muscular movement which emphasises speech. Pantomime is a method of communication in which spoken language is replaced by acting, and may include a series of gestures, each of which conveys a single meaning. Language includes all systems of communication, not only speech but the expression and understanding of written words, signs, gestures and music.

THE DEVELOPMENT OF SPEECH

It is important to realise firstly the comparatively late acquirement of speech in biological history (phylogenetic development), and secondly to understand how an individual person learns to speak (ontogenetic development).

Phylogenetic development

The age of the planet on which we live has been estimated as 2000 million years. Life in its earliest form occurred in about half that time, i.e. 1000 million years. An animal capable of making a noise (i.e. possessing a jointed larynx) came into existence 200 million years ago, but true and false vocal cords with the formation of a cochlea did not take place until perhaps 50 million years ago.

Although some animals, for example, the cock, hawk and rat make signals, and apes chatter and lions roar, these sounds are inborn, species-characteristic and limited to a specific reaction. The talking of parrots is mimicry and not speech in the scientific sense since there is no question of the bird formulating thoughts into words or understanding the sounds it utters. The 'language' of birds is in fact limited to communicating their desire for food, sexual needs, warnings of danger or mimicry, whereas human language covers an infinite number of thoughts, abstract as well as concrete. Questions can be asked and answered allowing an exchange of ideas and arguments, and humans also have the unique privilege of telling lies, believing or disbelieving. Although the faculty of speech is inborn, individual language has to be learnt.

There are several hypotheses as to how man acquired speech. Max Müller described the following: (1) the 'Ding-dong' theory—suggesting that there is an inherent connection between words and the things they stand for; (2) the 'Bow-wow' theory—suggesting that speech arose out of onomatopoeic sounds; (3) the 'Pooh-pooh' theory—indicating that by involuntary sounds and interjection, speech was acquired like the 'speech' of lower animals and birds; and (4) the 'Yo-heave-ho' theory—suggesting that man began to learn to speak from the sounds associated with communal physical effort. Early speech consisted of cries of emotion, e.g. fear, joy, anger and these corresponded to animal sound signals. Curses and exclamations lack the distinctive features of human speech since they may be uttered involuntarily and are automatic expressions of the emotions. Some of these interjections are conventially described as 'whew', 'ah', 'urgh', 'humph'.

The earliest man of which we have evidence (Java man) lived about one million years ago. A more developed creature (Heidelberg man) appeared half a million years ago, Neanderthal man about 150,000 years ago, and Cromagnon man about 50,000 years ago. Man began to speak as soon as he used tools (i.e. during the first Pleistocene period): the cooperation of individuals is needed both for speech and the use of tools and probably the first role of speech was to control behaviour.

Man did not give up his nomadic life and develop agriculture until 7000 B.C., whereas the first writing of which we have evidence is approximately 4000 B.C.: the Samarians of Mesopotamia were writing 3500 years before the birth of Christ. Speech then, is a recent development in the history of the world and its life.

Ontogenetic development of speech

Speech is acquired by the process of learning, which may be defined as the change in behaviour and perception of an organism as a consequence of its experience. A baby produces sound by crying as soon as it is born and, after a month, the cry becomes differentiated so that a mother appreciates its particular significance. As early as 2 months, an infant recognises the human voice, and soon after begins babbling: this is an essential part in the development of speech since it is a means of autostimulation (auditory feedback): the baby will stop babbling with any auditory stimulus—particularly if spoken to. At 6 months, the infant will distinguish between affectionate and scolding terms, and about this time the babbling becomes rhythmic (lalling). At about 9 months of age the child recognises familiar words and says 'Mama' and 'Dada'. It repeats words it hears—echolalia or psittacism, ('psittakos'—a parrot). The child loses nearly all the babbling sounds when it begins to articulate, and some children pass through a mute period between the babbling and language learning periods. In all languages, vowels are learned before consonants, the first vowel learned is an 'a', and the first consonant is an 'm'.

At 12 months of age, there will be a response to simple commands, and by 18 months the infant will acquire several words, many of which are peculiar to the child (idioglossia) but about 10–20 of these are meaningful. Although the learning of speech is relatively slow in the first 18 months, it is rapid for the next year, so that by the age of $2\frac{1}{2}$ years the child can say two-word phrases. The rate of learning slows off at the age of $2\frac{1}{2}$ years, the child acquiring about 500 new words each year and fully acquired speech—involved the use of sentences—comes gradually during the next few years.

The rapidity of learning depends not only on intelligence, but on the stimulation to speak, e.g. the home atmosphere and the social class of the parents. An only child is more likely to develop speech earlier than twins; the child of bilingual parents and a child in an orphanage are often slower than average.

The laborious learning of words, movements and reactions during early childhood depends on a system of repetitions and copying, trial and error. When the infant learns his first word, he has been listening to sounds of both himself and his mother; both use their personal pleasure as a facilitating mechanism, so that the sound is repeated in order to experience the pleasure again. When a child says 'Dada' he is repeating what he hears and then he correlates this with the seeing of a man; this necessitates remembering what the man looks like, and experiencing a feeling of familiarity and pleasure at the sight. The first process of repeating sounds soon becomes associated with the receptive systems, especially vision. The various sensations, including those from the muscles of the mouth and larynx, are essential for the registration of the neuronal patterns required to make the various noises that result in speech. The subsequent development of vocabulary and grammar is an elaboration of the more fundamental mechanism of registration. Learning to read and write, and correct spelling, involves many complex processes as does the capacity to name an object. Writing and reading are then learnt according to a programme and this capacity for learning is developed so that further knowledge can be superimposed. The neurological mechanisms depend partly on the repetition of previous responses; this is closely concerned with memory, which in its simplest form is the ability to repeat or recall a previous stimulus.

Animals learn to respond to sights, sounds and other sensations with motor reactions which may include making a noise; man has learned to produce a great variety of noises in relation to different objects, activities and feelings; in doing this, he uses highly specialised parts of his brain. Language and speech, as well as the related faculties of memory, learning and calculation are dependent on brain mechanisms which are integrated in, and controlled by, the cerebral hemispheres.

CHAPTER 2

THE BRAIN AND ITS FUNCTIONS

The brain is the most complicated organ of the body. It is composed of a complex network of nerve cells and fibres, requiring a rich blood supply (see Chapter 17) so that adequate oxygen, glucose, vitamins etc. are made available for metabolism. Restriction of these requirements will impair brain function and destruction of the nerve cells will lead to irreversible disorders.

Embryologically the anterior end of the central nervous system is modified into three parts, viz. the fore-brain, mid-brain and hind-brain. With development these parts increase in size and complexity, so that an adult human brain consists of many folded areas (gyri) with fissures in between (sulci). This convolutional pattern enables man to have the maximum amount of cerebral cortex in the smallest possible volume.

The surface of the brain (cortex) comprises the grey matter, which contains the nerve *cells* (neurones). This covers the underlying white matter which consists mainly of nerve *fibres*. In addition to the nerve cells and their fibres, the brain substance also contains connective tissue cells. These are of three types: astrocytes, oligodendrocytes and microglia. There are also aggregations of neurones (nuclei) forming the basal ganglia which lie in the depths of each cerebral hemisphere. The cerebral hemispheres are joined together by the corpus callosum and each is connected with the brain stem by the cerebral peduncles. The brain stem has three parts: mid-brain, pons and medulla (or bulb).

The cerebellum consists of right and left cerebellar hemispheres, joined in the mid line by the vermis. Each cerebellar hemisphere is connected to the corresponding side of the brain stem by three cere-bellar peduncles: superior (brachium conjunctivum), middle (brachium pontis) and inferior (restiform body).

Each cerebral hemisphere consists of frontal, parietal, temporal and occipital lobes (see Fig. 1). The central (Rolandic) fissure separates the frontal from the parietal lobe. The lateral (Sylvian) fissure demarcates the upper part of the temporal lobe. The occipital lobe is the posterior part of the hemisphere, containing the calcarine (visual) cortex. Many

LATERAL SURFACE OF CEREBRAL HEMISPHERE

FIGURE I. Diagram of the lateral surface of the left cerebral hemisphere.

of the main gyri are named and the whole cortex has been divided into anatomical regions, numbered as Brodmann's areas.

The phrenologists considered that the fissures divided the brain into regions which were concerned with personality characteristics, for example, intelligence, memory and piety. These attempts to localise specific function to certain anatomical areas conflicted with the view that the brain was an amorphous organ whose cells, like the cells of the liver, could function in many capacities. Localisation of speech function within the brain was suggested by Broca in 1861, and subsequent observations including experiments using electrical stimulation have shown that other important functions are controlled by specific parts of the brain. Thus the cerebral control of movements is located in the precentral gyrus which is the main motor area. The postcentral gyrus represents sensory functions; the visual cortex is in the occipital lobe. There are also so-called non-committed areas of the brain, for example in the frontal lobes, containing association fibres so that the brain can function as a whole.

THE SPEECH AREA

The surface markings of the area of the dominant cerebral hemisphere controlling speech and language functions are shown in Fig. 2. This includes the lowermost part of the pre-central gyrus (Broca's area) and post-central gyrus, the supramarginal and angular gyri, the inferior parietal gyri and upper part of the temporal lobe (Wernicke's area). The disorders of speech due to lesions in this area are described in Chapter 9. The concept of *cerebral dominance* is discussed in Chapter 5.

FIGURE 2. The thick line indicates the limits of the area of the brain within which a small wound will cause aphasia (Russell W.R. 1963). The speech area thus lies within this and includes Broca's and Wernicke's areas. (Reproduced by permission of the author and the *Lancet*.)

THE FRONTAL LOBES

The pre-central gyrus in each cerebral hemisphere contains the motor cortex, in which the large motor nerve cells (Betz cells) are situated. The face is represented by the lower-most part in the inferior frontal region, there is a large area for the hand and upper limb in the middle, and the leg area is uppermost (viz. in the parasagittal region) and extends over the medial surface of the hemisphere. The area anterior to the pre-central gyrus is called the pre-motor cortex, which covers a large association area for co-ordination of motor function.

Fibres from the motor cells of all parts of the motor cortex (see Fig. 3) penetrate the depths of the cerebral hemisphere in the corona

FIGURE 3. Diagram of upper and lower neurones. (Redrawn from *Neurology for Nurses*, by E.R. Bickerstaff, English Universities Press, London, 1965.)

radiata, coming closer together to pass through the internal capsule; this lies between the lenticular nucleus laterally and the caudate nucleus and thalamus medially. In the internal capsule, the fibres subserving the face area are in the front, the leg area posteriorly and the arm and trunk fibres in between. The fibres then descend through the cerebral peduncles, mid-brain and pons. In the brain stem most of the cortico-*bulbar* fibres decussate and terminate in synapses (see page 58) with the *motor nuclei of the cranial nerves*. Likewise the majority of cortico-*spinal* fibres decussate to form the pyramids, and then descend in the lateral columns of the spinal cord as the pyramidal (cortico-spinal) tracts, terminating in synapses with the *anterior horn cells of the spinal cord*. This is the first part of the motor pathway, the upper motor neurone (U.M.N.). It thus extends from the motor cells of the frontal cortex, either via the cortico-bulbar fibres to the synapses with the cells of the motor nuclei of the cranial nerves in the medulla, or via the cortico-spinal fibres to the synapses with the anterior horn cells of the spinal cord. The upper motor neurones transmit the impulses from the cerebral hemispheres which initiate, associate and control voluntary and automatic muscular action and reaction. They are linked in the cerebral hemispheres by the association areas with the other parts of the brain which receive the sensory, visual and auditory stimuli. Integration of stimuli received by, and emanating from, all parts of the brain allows co-ordinated physical and mental reactions, and the separation of functions for the purpose of description is artificial. It may also be fallacious to draw conclusions about the normal functioning of the brain from a study of the effects of damage to localised areas. (Comparison can be made with an electrical circuit where damage to the battery or generating system will have an effect on all points and connections, whereas damage to a single wire will have very different effects depending upon its situation in the circuit and its relation to other points, for example, whether connected in series or parallel.)

Bilateral representation

Not all the cortico-bulbar and cortico-spinal (upper motor neurone) fibres cross to the opposite side of the brain stem and spinal cord, a small proportion remaining uncrossed. Thus some of the motor nuclei in the brain stem have bilateral cerebral representation and, if the crossing fibres from one hemisphere are damaged, function may be maintained by the uncrossed fibres from the unaffected side. This explains why in many hemiplegic patients only the lower part of the face is affected and there is no paralysis of the upper part of the face, nor of the palate or tongue. For further details about this, see Chapter 10.

Other frontal lobe functions

Personality, temperament, emotional control and behaviour are dependent upon mechanisms in the frontal lobes, and these may become disturbed if either or both of the frontal lobes become damaged or diseased. The frontal lobes are often considered to be the seat of the mind and intelligence, but intellectual function is dependent upon integration of the whole cerebral cortex. Normal behaviour depends largely on a balance between initiative and self control, and the ability to act appropriately has come to be part of everyday life and social necessity. The primitive instincts of a child normally become inhibited by conditioning and, with maturity, customs and etiquette are learnt so that impulses, emotions and actions are suppressed to conform with the requirements of the environment.

Voluntary control of movements of the head and neck and eye movements are also associated with frontal lobe function, as is control of the bladder and sexual functions.

Frontal lobe syndromes

Patients with frontal lobe disorders manifest disinhibition, with inadequately controlled, aggressive or anti-social behaviour, as well as dementia (see Chapter 15), deterioration of personality and intellect, slowness of thought and loss of initiative. The mental changes resulting from frontal lobe lesions include defects of emotional control; there is a tendency to laugh childishly or inappropriately, with inability to realise the true seriousness of situations, for example, lack of insight into the gravity of medical disability. Changes in mood range from the feeling of well-being or excessive cheerfulness (euphoria) which is inappropriate and pathological, to mania; alternatively the patient becomes depressed, miserable and melancholic without adequate reason.

Lessions in the motor area will cause weakness in the opposite side of the body, i.e. the face, arm or leg, according to the situation and extent of the lesion. The terms *hemiparesis* or *hemiplegia* are used to describe respectively weakness or paralysis of one half of the body (i.e. face, arm and leg); *monoplegia* means paralysis of one limb, either arm or leg (see Chapter 10).

THE PARIETAL LOBES

The parietal lobes are the main receiving areas for sensory impulses and stimuli. Parts of the body are represented in the contralateral sensory cortex of the post-central gyrus in the same way as on the motor side. The sensory impulses travel from the end organs in the skin, mucles, joints and other tissues of the body and are conveyed proximally in centripetal fashion via the sensory (spinal and cranial) nerves. From the dorsal root ganglia, the fibres of the posterior nerve roots enter the spinal cord and form the main sensory tracts, which pass up via the brain stem to the first receiving station in the thalamus. The impulses are then relayed from the thalamus through the posterior part of the internal capsule and radiate out to the appropriate parts of the sensory cortex.

Basic sensations such as touch pass to the post-central gyrus, whereas impulses for finer discrimination and interpretation pass to the large area of the parietal lobe posterior to the post-central gyrus. These finer discriminative functions are concerned with size, shape and consistency of substances which are felt and allow differentiation of complicated sensations, appreciation of the sense of position of the opposite side of the body, and the location of particular parts of the body in space. This is a highly developed function which becomes automatic, so that the position and movement of a hand is known both in relation to a given object and also in relation to other parts of the body. Orientation in space and appreciation of the body-image (see page 25) are dependent upon the function of the association areas of the parietal region. These are linked with the visual cortex in the occipital region and performance of many manoeuvres is improved by seeing.

Parietal lobe syndromes

Damage to the sensory pathways or receiving areas in one parietal lobe will cause a contralateral hemianaesthesia, i.e. impairment of sensation on the opposite side of the body. If the lesion is localised, the sensory loss may be limited—e.g. to the hand or leg. Parietal lobe lesions may also cause various types of apraxia and agnosia, disoreintation and disturbances of the body image (see Chapter 4) and a homonymous hemianopia if the optic radiation is involved (see page 13).

THE TEMPORAL LOBES

A large part of the temporal lobe of the dominant cerebral hemisphere is concerned with speech, particularly the middle zone of the upper temporal convolution (Wernicke's area). This forms part of the main auditory-receptive centre for the assimilation and interpretation of sounds required for the understanding of speech. The medial part of each temporal lobe includes the uncus, hippocampus and amygdaloid body which are concerned with the senses of *smell and taste* and with *memory* (see Chapter 3). The hippocampus is linked with the mamillary bodies (corpora mamillaria) via the fornix of the corpus callosum, which also forms a connection with the hippocampus of the opposite temporal lobe.

Lesions confined to the temporal lobe cause no motor or sensory changes on the opposite side of the body but may involve the optic radiation and produce contralateral homonymous visual field defects (see Fig. 4). The anterior 5–6 cm of one temporal lobe can be removed surgically (temporal lobectomy) without any obvious clinical sequelae.

THE OCCIPITAL LOBES

These contain the calcarine (visual) cortex. A complete lesion on one side will give a homonymous hemianopia on the opposite side (see Fig. 4 (c)). Partial lesions of one occipital lobe will cause congruous defects or scotomata in the homonymous visual fields of various shapes, according to the exact extent of the lesion.

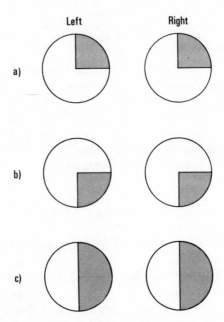

FIGURE 4. Visual field defects (represented by shaded areas):
     (a) right homonymous upper quadrantic
     (b) right homonymous lower quadrantic
     (c) right homonymous hemianopia

THE OPTIC RADIATION

The fibres forming this part of the visual pathway lie deep in the temporal and parietal lobes and convey impulses from the lateral geniculate body on each side to the visual cortex in the occipital lobe. A lesion of the temporal lobe may initially involve the lower part of the optic radiation as it passes round the temporal horn of the lateral ventricle and so cause contralateral homonymous *upper* quadrantic visual field defects (see Fig. 4 (a)). A lesion of the parietal lobe may involve the upper part of the optic radiation and so cause contralateral homonymous *lower* quadrantic visual field defects (see Fig. 4 (b)). If either temporal or parietal lobe lesions extend to involve the whole of the optic radiation, then a complete contralateral homonymous hemianopia will result (see Fig. 4 (c)).

CHAPTER 3
MEMORY AND AMNESIA

In addition to the functions of the brain described in the previous chapter, brain activity is reflected by the state of consciousness, which includes awareness, both of oneself and the environment, as well as the capacity to think, learn, speak and control behaviour. An essential common factor for the optimum performance of these functions is the ability to remember. Memory is the capacity to retain experiences and skills and involves reception, registration, retention, recall and reproduction. Each of these processes can be affected independently; for example, reception and registration can be left intact although other aspects of memory are disordered.

Non-specific mechanisms, such as attention and perception, are involved in reception so that memorising is less efficient when the individual is tired or emotionally upset or if attention is distracted by competing stimuli, for example, extraneous noise. The urge to remember depends greatly on the stimulus of interest together with the influence of the emotions such as joy, fear, love and hate. Motivation and concentration also act as important facilitating factors for memorising and successful learning. The word 'memory' is sometimes restricted to the recall of stored material, which is used with ever increasing confidence as the individual matures. Undoubtedly memory mechanisms have an important role in the development of verbal skills, intelligence, mathematical ability etc., but physiological mechanisms underlying the simplest memory, such as remembering how to walk, are little understood.

An essential part of the physiology of memory is the capacity to repeat previous responses and establish stores of neuronal patterns. Memories have been described as 'facilitated neuronal circuits which never rest'. Repetitive activity probably results in a lower threshold at synapses (see page 58) so that interneuronal communication, dependent on physico-chemical changes, becomes more efficient. There are probably separate biochemical mechanisms facilitating short-term and long-term memory, short-term memory being accompanied by structural changes in protein whereas long-term memory is associated with protein synthesis and is more stable than short-term memory. Conditioning of animals produces molecular changes within neurones as evidenced by an increased rate of R.N.A. (ribonucleic acid) neuronal synthesis; conversely, pharmacological inhibition of protein synthesis within the nerve cell can impair the processes of conditioning and learning.

Knowledge and capacity for thought are closely linked with memory for names, words, languages and music, and these are probably stored in the cortex and association areas of the temporal lobe, whereas memory for the motor and sensory skills seems to be a function of the frontal and parietal lobes. All these may be disorganised in lesions causing aphasia (Chapter 9) which may also interfere with the activity of the system whereby memories are preserved. Thought is of little avail without the retention of knowledge, and both recently acquired and long established memories are important for each facet of the speech mechanism, whether it be of sound, sight, the capacity to make a remembered noise in speaking, or movement in writing. It is in this way that the formulation of thoughts and their transfer into words, as well as the ability to learn and judge, have to be integrated with memories derived from events heard and seen.

Many people depend on visual memory, and use of the storage systems is also required when reading. This process includes recognition of the visual patterns of the letters and words and of the associations which add a 'meaning' to the words (although we have little knowledge of what meaning involves in physiological terms). Reading also demands the capacity to remember what is read for long enough to correlate it with later pages. The inability to remember what has been read might be due to a lesion either of the hippocampus or of the storage mechanisms in the posterior parietal lobes.

Retention (the storage of memory) includes organisation and integration and can be improved voluntarily, for example by repetition. Recall is the process by which stored memories are brought into consciousness, usually with voluntary effort. Defective recall is usually associated with defective retention and patients may attempt to fill in the gaps in their memory by confabulation, an example of abnormal behaviour accompanying many amnestic states.

Papez (1973) suggested a circuit as the basis for memory integration; this consisted of Ammon's horn, the fornix cerebri, the mamillary bodies, the bundle of Vicq d'Azyr, the anterior thalamic nuclei and the cingulum; between the cingulum and the hippocampal gyrus there are further connections.

The fornix cerebri is the main efferent pathway from the hippocampal gyrus to the mamillary body, but there are fibres in the fornix that arise in other structures and it is estimated that only one-third of the two million fibres in the fornix reaches the mamillary bodies. Although interruption of the Papez circuit has been used to explain defects of memory, this is an over-simplification since bilateral interruption of the circuit need not produce a permanent memory defect; nor does this theory explain memory loss seen in frontal and occipital lesions. Other parts of the brain such as the reticular formation are also concerned in memory function since a state of alertness is important for learning.

Although the *fronto-hypothalamic* system contributes to the emotional drive to remember, it is the *fronto-temporal* neuronal system, particularly in the dominant hemisphere, which facilitates the highly elaborate activity that provides the memory required for speech, thought, initiative and the general control of behaviour. The cortical connections with the thalamus and with the opposite cerebral hemisphere via the corpus callosum are also important so that lesions of these deeply situated structures may also lead to severe disorganisation.

Recently acquired memories are formed from information reaching the sensory receiving areas including the visual and auditory cortex, and there is evidence to suggest that the hippocampus, the fornix of the corpus callosum and the mamillary bodies form a facilitating mechanism for the storage of current events and for the learning of new material. Old established memories on the other hand appear to depend on a different mechanism, maintained by the spontaneous activity of neurones, which is less vulnerable to degenerative and other disease processes. Thus the activity of the hippocampal system which facilitates the storage of current events tends to decline in old age, and this accounts for the forgetfulness of old people who fail to remember day-to-day happenings yet refer accurately to long past events.

Since conscious recall involves using a small sample from a vast mass of experience, most of which have been forgotten, the physiology of forgetting is a relevant consideration. Fogetting is the failure of voluntary recall and may be due to emotional repression; it is probably not a failure to learn but an active process of learning not to remember. Forgotten memories can be shown to be present by the phenomena of dreams, hypnosis, and analysis.

Ribot (1882) first postulated the law of regression in which the ease of retrieval of memories varies inversely with their recency, as happens in normal forgetting—the longer the time since an event occurred the more likely it is to be forgotten. The amount remembered drops steeply in the first few seconds and then levels out, but more is forgotten in the first few minutes after an event than in subsequent periods. Ribot also listed successive stages in loss of content; for example, events were first forgotten, then ideas, then feelings and, last of all, actions. In language, proper names were forgotten first, then common nouns, then adjectives, then interjections, and finally gestures. In effect, emotional appreciation in art goes first, then ambition and, last of all, fear and anger. This suggests that there is a gradient from the complex to the simple and from the voluntary to the involuntary.

The clinical assessment of memory is obtained by tests of immediate, short-term and long-term memory.

Immediate memory can be assessed clinically by digit span; normally six digits can be repeated forward and five digits backwards. The Babcock sentence: "There is one thing a nation must have to be rich and great, and that is a large, secure supply of wood", can normally be repeated word perfect after three attempts. The span of immediate memory is from 30 seconds to 1 minute and it is characterised by a limited capacity. Disorders of immediate memory produce a failure to retain ongoing events, i.e. anterograde amnesia. Loss of immediate memory can produce disorientation in time and space and, if insight is absent, paranoia.

Short-term memory can be tested by the 'hidden' objects' test (in which familiar objects are hidden and 15 minutes later the patient is asked to find them), the capacity for remembering playing cards, and by the 'name, address and flower' test. Whereas immediate memory concerns a span of seconds, recent and short-term memory has a span of hours or days. Short-term memories are easily recalled, rapidly forgotten and without permanent record. When short-term memory is normal, registration cannot be at fault.

Long-term memory relates to remote events of a few months or many years ago and has a larger capacity and slower forgetting, being the basis of past learning. When there is a disturbance of long-term memory, it is difficult to decide whether this is due to failure of retention or failure of recall. Since there is no alteration of consciousness, these amnestic syndromes can be distinguished from confusional states.

Mechanisms of short-term and long-term memory are distinct and differentially susceptible to clinical conditions. This is evident from the striking loss of the ability to store current events while remote memories are conserved, as seen not only in old age as already mentioned, but also in organic brain diseases, particularly with bilateral lesions or after excision of the temporal lobes.

AMNESIA

Amnesia (loss of memory) may be caused by a variety of disorders affecting the brain. Memory impairment is often the first manifestation of a progressive dementia (see Chapter 15). However, many of the following conditions which cause amnesia recover spontaneously or are reversible with appropriate treatment.

Trauma

Amnesia mainly for recent events, and confusion of thought are features of concussion resulting from a head injury (see Chapter 19). In addition to post-traumatic amnesia (P.T.A.), there may also be loss of memory for a period of time leading up to and immediately preceding the impact, and this is called retrograde amnesia (R.A.). Concussion is due to brain damage which is not macroscopically visible and the resultant amnesia may be due to disturbance of neuronal molecules since, experimentally, concussed guinea pigs show alterations in Nissl substance (which contains R.N.A.). A longer period of P.T.A. occurs with lesions of the dominant left temporal lobe as compared with lesions of the right temporal lobe and other parts of the brain. The ability to remember is regained when hippocampal function recovers or if the hippocampus of the opposite hemisphere takes over.

ECT

Amnesia may occur after electroconvulsive therapy (E.C.T.) which is given for the treatment of depression, and recovery is similar to that seen in post-traumatic cases. Orientation in place occurs before orientation in time and the longest established memories are the first to recover. Names learned early in life return before those acquired later. Short-term memory and the ability to learn new material usually return within 2–3 weeks, but some deficit may persist for several months. This effect on memory can be prevented or reduced by applying the electric shock unilaterally to the non-dominant cerebral hemisphere.

Encephalopathy

Persistent loss of memory for recent events with retrograde amnesia for months, but retention of memory for long-past events has been reported following *encephalitis* (Rose and Symonds, 1960). In this series the patients were unable to remember anything of a current experience even for a space of a few minutes, yet did not show confabulation. One of the 4 cases in the series has died, and autopsy revealed bilateral atrophy of the temporal lobes.

Local and diffuse brain infections due to various types of encephalitis and tuberculous meningitis (see Chapter 18) can also cause periodic confusion and amnesia which usually clear with recovery from the infection.

Transient amnesia may occur in any severe infection, for example with septicaemia and pneumonia and, on recovery, the patient may have no recollection of the acute state of the illness. Loss of memory and a confusional state may last for minutes or hours and be followed by complete recovery.

Similar transient disturbances may be due to *metabolic disorders*, for example hepatic, renal or respiratory failure, deficiency diseases, drugs and other toxic substances—classic examples being acute alcoholic poisoning and bromide intoxication.

Korsakoff's psychosis and/or *Wernicke's encephalopathy*, often accompanied by peripheral neuropathy, may result from chronic alcoholism which induces deficiency of thiamine and other vitamins of the B group.

Features of the syndrome described by Korsakoff (1887) include loss of memory for recent events, confabulation, confusion with disorientation in time and space, false recognition, lack of insight, and apathy. Vocabulary and previously acquired skills are usually preserved and remote memory, although impaired, is better than recent memory. Characteristic of Korsakoff's psychosis is the impaired ability to acquire new information—anterograde amnesia. Immediate memory is normal but short-term memory is poor and, on psychometric testing, there is an atypical learning curve with frequent perseveration. Confabulation is frequent in response to questions rather than spontaneous. It is either entirely imaginary or dependent on partial recollections; answers are consistent with the patient's usual activities and occupation but tend to change from one day to the next and consist of 'pseudo-reminiscences' (false memories of familiar happenings).

Wernicke's encephalopathy also begins with a global confusional state evidenced by drowsiness, inattention, and disorientation with failure of identification. Nystagmus is nearly always present and ocular palsy, usually incomplete, is present in the majority and delirium tremens in about one-third of cases.

Early treatment with thiamine usually leads to rapid improvement, although the mental disturbances tend to recover only slowly. Amnesia persists for the period of the illness with difficulty in learning and memorising. Retrograde amnesia is rarely complete, the patient retaining islands of information but there is 'telescoping' in which long-past events are thought of as occurring more recently; this incorrect sequencing may partly account for confabulation together with the lack of insight into the amnesia and the associated disorder of perception. In fatal cases the main post-mortem findings are focal areas of haemorrhage and neuronal degeneration in the mamillary bodies and mid-brain.

Transient Global Amnesia

Transient global amnesia is an organic syndrome in which acute disorientation with amnesia of sudden onset lasts for a few hours, although perception and personal identity are preserved. Usually there is complete recovery with a retrograde amnesia that shrinks, although memory of events during the episode does not return. The cause is probably bilateral temporal lobe ischaemia involving the hippocampal regions.

Epilepsy

Transient amnesia is an inevitable component of any attack of loss of consciousness or awareness and so occurs in epilepsy (see Chapter 14). Petit mal consists of transient loss of awareness with amnesia of only seconds after which the child immediately resumes activity or conversation. Retrograde amnesia after a grand mal fit may obliterate the aura and there may also be a period of post-ictal amnesia with confusion and automatism (inappropriate, fragmented or repetitive behaviour of which the patient later has no memory).

Although post-ictal amnesia *per se* has no localising significance, automatism is often associated with a focus in the medial part of temporal lobe. Attacks of temporal lobe epilepsy often involve some memory disturbance, a minority have the classical aura of déjà vu (a sensation of familiarity) or jamais vu (a sensation of strangeness) and the various hallucinations which may also occur can be regarded as forced or distorted memories. These features of temporal lobe attacks mimic or reflect the normal facilitating mechanisms, the epileptic activity stimulating the storage systems concerned with the special senses in the hippocampus.

Hysteria

Hysterical amnesia tends to occur in stressful situations, such as domestic disharmony or failure at work. The distinction between this and other forms of amnesia is that the capacity to recall memories still remains, as can be proven using various techniques such as hypnosis or narco-analysis. Although the memories are beyond voluntary recall they can occur in dreams, or influence behaviour. Hysterical amnesia commonly consists of a 'fugue' lasting for a few hours or even days during which the individual either wanders around aimlessly or makes a specific journey apparently without any sense of identity. Occasionally there is an alternating amnesia in which different episodes are remembered alternately suggesting a 'multiple personality' syndrome. As in normal forgetting, there is resistance to remembering unpleasant events; hysterical amnesia, although subconscious, serves as a defence mechanism and is often associated with anxiety and depression. Recovery, which can either be gradual or sudden, is usually spontaneous, for example when a relative appears, and is frequently associated with a feeling of exhilaration. Hypnosis is only partially successful.

CHAPTER 4
APRAXIA AND AGNOSIA

APRAXIA

The ability to perform purposeful movements and complicated skills is gradually learned by practice and experience; these motor activities are organised and stored by the association areas of the frontal and parietal lobes. Apraxia is the loss of skill required for complex actions due to inability to perform specific movements at will, yet the same movements can be performed in isolation or involuntarily. There is no paralysis and the individual muscles can participate in other movements. The causative lesion involves the relevant association areas representing movements rather than individual muscles, and interferes with the control of movements by the corresponding part of the motor cortex, although the fibres forming the main motor pathway remain intact.

In general, the more recently acquired actions are lost first, so that in mild cases the less complicated and primitive skills are preserved. In severe forms the patient regresses to a state comparable to infancy with inco-ordinate movements affecting actions such as walking or standing. These movements, automatic in adult life, are based on the concept of 'kinetic engrams' and the disturbances of these have been called limb-kinetic, innervatory or cortical apraxia.

Ideomotor apraxia is the term suggested when the kinetic engrams are present, the patient has no difficulty in formulating the idea of the act which he wishes to carry out but finds himself unable to execute it. Simple tests such as asking a patient to salute, make a fist or shake hands, reveal an ideomotor apraxia whereas other movements such as grasping an object can be done automatically.

Ideational apraxia is when the conception of the movement is faulty, for example, on being asked to light a cigarette, the patient puts the match into his mouth instead of the cigarette. This type is closely linked with ideomotor apraxia and agnosia as there is clearly a failure to recognise the nature or use of the object for which the movements are required. In severe forms, ideational apraxia is combined with ideomotor apraxia.

There may also be an inability to dress or undress (*dressing apraxia*), construct models from blocks or letters with matches (*constructional apraxia*).

With regard to speech, apraxia of the lips or tongue is relatively common and will produce an *articulatory apraxia* (apraxic dysarthria), automatic movements of the tongue and facial muscles being preserved. Facial apraxia is not uncommonly associated with expressive and nominal aphasia. Constructional apraxia may interfere with drawing or writing, and is thus a cause of dysgraphia which may be distinguishable from that resulting from a specific defect of language.

Although apraxia is manifest as a motor disability, there is often an element of agnosia as well; in dressing apraxia, the patient may be unable to relate the spatial forms of his garments to that of his body, and in constructional apraxia the patient may be unaware of the inadequacy of his achievement and so there may be defective recognition both of the model and the copy.

The site of the lesion causing apraxia is usually the post-central area of the parietal lobe but the temporal lobe is sometimes involved. Lesions causing ideational and ideomotor apraxia are usually bilateral but constructional apraxia may be caused by a lesion in either hemisphere, and dressing apraxia by a lesion of the non-dominant hemisphere.

AGNOSIA

The ability to interpret sensory stimuli which are conveyed to the brain from the special senses (e.g. visual and auditory) and from other parts of the body (e.g. touch) is a function of the cerebral hemispheres. The cortex of the temporal, parietal and occipital lobes are mainly concerned with the processes of recognition or perception of sensory stimuli (gnosis). This implies that the crude sensory stimuli acquire significance by collation with previous experiences stored as memories in the appropriate association areas.

Agnosia, a term first introduced by Freud in 1891, means a loss of this ability to recognise these sensory experiences; it is a defect of perception due to a disorder of cerebral mechanisms. The lesions causing the defects involve localised areas of the cerebral cortex and their association areas, the primary sensory pathways being intact. The various types of agnosia depend on the sensory modality involved.

Visual Agnosia

Visual agnosia was called 'imperception' by Hughlings Jackson and various types are now described.

Visual object agnosia is the inability to recognise objects seen, this failure not being attributable to defects of vision or to general intellectual impairment. Not only is there failure to recognise an object but also what the object is used for (cf: nominal aphasia, in which the object cannot be named but its nature or use can often be described). A patient with visual agnosia is usually able to name the object if allowed to feel it. The lesion responsible for visual object agnosia is thought to be in the cortex of the 2nd and 3rd occipital convolutions or possibly in the splenium of the corpus callosum, through which pass fibres linking the visual cortex of the two hemispheres.

Visual object agnosia is sometimes associated with tactile agnosia, alexia, constructional apraxia and Gerstmann's syndrome (see page 26).

Dyslexia (see Chapters 6 and 9) may also be a type of visual agnosia, when the patterns produced by letters, words, numbers or music fail to be recognised or understood. The meaning must be stored in order to obtain the sequence of what follows. A homonymous hemianopia due to lesions of the optic radiation may also cause difficulty with reading; but the difficulties due to defects of the visual fields and of visual acuity differ from dyslexia which concerns the problems of using and understanding visual symbol patterns. The visual pathways of the brain play a large part in language, learning, memory and thought; congenitally blind patients develop speech mechanisms differently (Critchley, 1953).

Spelling difficulties may also be due to disturbances of visual imagery due to lesions in the posterior parietal region.

Many other types of visual agnosia have been described. *Prosopagnosia* is a name given to the failure to recognise faces, normally well-known. *Simultanagnosia* is the failure to appreciate the meaning of a complex picture or recognise a combination of details although the individual elements are correctly recognised. This is also called visual extinction and indicates a lesion of the posterior temporal or parietal lobe. Visual inattention is the failure to see an object on one side when shown objects on both sides of the visual field simultaneously, there being no defect when each object is shown separately. *Agnosia for colours* has to be distinguished from nominal aphasia in which the colours are recognised but cannot be named. *Visual disorientation* may include defective visual localisation, loss of visual imagery, loss of stereoscopic vision and spatial agnosia. *Loss of topographical memory* may also occur independently of other forms of visual disorientation and of loss of memory for objects.

Auditory Agnosia

In auditory agnosia, hearing is not impaired but there is an inability to recognise or distinguish the sounds which are heard due to a lesion of the left superior temporal convolution. With the eyes closed or covered, the patient cannot recognise familiar noises, such as the jingling of keys or coins. The loss of recognition of musical sounds is called *sensory amusia*. Failure to understand spoken speech (word deafness or receptive aphasia) may also be a form of auditory agnosia.

Tactile Agnosia

Tactile agnosia, the failure to recognise objects by touch, is also called *astereognosis*. Sensation in the hands is otherwise normal, but the patient fails to recognise the shape, size or consistency of the object, which is placed in his hand without his being allowed to see it. Tactile agnosia may occur without visual agnosia, so that patients can then recognise by sight what they cannot recognise by feel. The lesion responsible is thought to be in the supramarginal gyrus of the parietal lobe, and there is evidence that in right handed persons bilateral tactile agnosia may be produced by a lesion in this area of the left cerebral hemisphere, suggesting that there may be dominance for tactile recognition.

The body image

The perception and recognition of movements of all parts of our body both in relation to each other and to the external environment are integrated so that we develop a body schema or awareness of our body image. Learning and memory mechanisms allow the use of previous experiences so that mental and physical performances become automatic or can be geared to changes in oneself or in the environment.

This concept of the body image implies that a storage, collating and selecting system exists in the association areas, particularly of the parietal lobes.

Somatagnosia is the name given to disorders of the body schema; these include imperception or neglect of parts of the body (*auto-topagnosia*) right-left disorientation (i.e. the inability to distinguish right from left) and denial of disability, e.g. unawareness of a hemiplegic limb (*anosognosia*). Another example is seen in some patients with complete cortical blindness who deny that they are blind but confabulate that they can see (*Anton's syndrome*).

The variety of possible defects, single and combined, is considerable. One such combination is *Gerstmann's syndrome*, viz: finger agnosia (an inability of the patient to recognise or identify his own fingers or those of the observer) right-left disorientation, agraphia and acalculia.

Site of lesions causing Agnosia

Gerstmann's syndrome results from a lesion of the left supra-marginal and angular gyri, but there is controversy as to whether this is a distinct entity or merely represents one of a variety of combined defects resulting from lesions of the parietal cortex. Unilateral spatial agnosia and prosopagnosia are usually due to a parieto-occipital lesion of the non-dominant hemisphere. In other types of agnosia the lesions are usually extensive and may be bilateral but we cannot say that there is an exact anatomical localisation for each type of agnosia.

CHAPTER 5
CEREBRAL DOMINANCE

The cerebral hemisphere controlling speech is called the dominant hemisphere, and the concept of cerebral dominance is closely related to the problems of aphasia. Bouillard in 1865 suggested that cerebral dominance for speech and handedness were in some way interconnected and later Hughlings Jackson introduced his concept of the 'leading hemisphere', implying a physiological rather than any anatomical difference between the two hemispheres. However recent studies have shown that the dominant parietal lobe controlling speech, spatial orientation and praxis is slightly larger and contains more nerve cells than the non-dominant parietal lobe. Furthermore the electro-encephalogram (see page 100) often shows a lower voltage alpha rhythm over the dominant hemisphere. Nevertheless there is some evidence that the non-dominant right hemisphere may also possess some limited language capacity in right-handed adults, being concerned more with verbal comprehension than with verbal expression (Gazzaniga and Hillyard, 1971).

Laterality implies that one side is preferred when performing certain skills, for example with the hand, foot or eye. Usually there is consistence in the side preferred for a particular skill but laterality depends upon the skill tested, e.g. a person may write with the left hand and throw a ball with the right, yet prefer to kick a ball with the left foot; this is called mixed laterality or mixed dominance. Although there may be a preferred eye, e.g. in looking through a telescope or kaleidoscope, this cannot be directly related to cerebral dominance since the nerve fibres from each eye go to both hemispheres. To test visual dominance, the choice of left or right visual fields would have to be tested. The relationship between eyedness and cerebral dominance may also depend upon which hand is preferred for holding the telescope.

Right-handedness is a feature of the majority of people in all nations and such evidence as is available, e.g. from prehistoric cave paintings, suggests that this has always been so. It is not known for certain whether dextrality is an organic or cultural heritage—even the accepted familial trend of sinistrality is unhelpful since this could be either genetic or environmental (or both).

An infant does not show any preference for either hand until the age of about 9 months when speech begins. Handedness slowly becomes established—with speech—after the age of two, and laterality is undoubtedly governed in some cases by agenesis or damage of one cerebral hemisphere. It is now generally recognised that there are varying degrees of laterality, some people being more strongly right-handed than others. True ambidexterity, i.e. the ability to use either hand equally well, is probably quite rare.

It used to be thought that the left cerebral hemisphere was dominant for speech in right handers and the right hemisphere in left-handers. However in 1959 Penfield and Roberts concluded from studies of cortical stimulation and excision in patients with epilepsy that the left cerebral hemisphere was dominant for speech in nearly everyone, whether left-handed or right-handed, provided that one excluded cases of pathological left-handedness, i.e. due to trauma or disease of the left hemisphere at birth or during infancy. The present position regarding the relationship between cerebral dominance and handedness is that the left cerebral hemisphere is almost always dominant for speech in right-handers with very rare exceptions. In left-handers the pattern of cerebral dominance for language functions is more complex (Zangwill, 1967; Wyke, 1971). The left cerebral hemisphere is also dominant for speech in a proportion (probably 50%) of left-handers. There are other left-handers whose right cerebral hemisphere is dominant and in these cases there is by no means always evidence of trauma or disease to the left hemisphere at birth or during infancy. Confirmation of this view has been obtained from the study of brain wounds (Russell and Espir, 1961) and cases of post-traumatic epilepsy having an aphasic aura (see Chapter 14) and also from the technique of intracarotid arterial injection (Milner, Branch and Rasmussen, 1964). It is also possible that in some cases both hemispheres may contribute to language functions without definite dominance on one side; this is the concept of *cerebral ambilaterality* suggested by Zangwill (1960).

Left-handedness

Left-handed subjects are those who prefer to use the left hand for the performance of the majority of one-handed motor skills, e.g. throwing a ball and using a racquet; this may include preference for kicking a ball with the left foot. The incidence of left-handedness in the general population ranges from 5 to 10%. It may be thought that left-handers who write with the left hand are more strongly left-handed than left-handers who write with the right hand and that they would be more likely to have the right hemisphere dominant or perhaps have cerebral ambilaterality; but whether a left-hander uses his left or right hand for writing does not necessarily indicate which hemisphere is dominant. Thus some left-handers who write with the left hand are rendered aphasic from left hemisphere lesions, and others, also left-handed writers, are rendered aphasic from right hemisphere lesions; the same applies to left-handers who write with the right hand.

Individual variation in the degree of laterality is common amongst left-handers, and many use their right hand more often and more skilfully than right-handers use their left.

CHAPTER 6
DEVELOPMENTAL SPEECH AND LANGUAGE DISORDERS

The development of a function depends upon learning processes which necessitate not only the making of new physiological pathways but also the inhibition of irrelevant responses, both at physiological and psychological levels. Learning to read and write involves organising a wide variety of perceptual experiences and motor responses, which may be interfered with by bodily disturbances or brain lesions. In the case of language function, the child has to learn to use these skills for the expression of his own feelings. The learning process is not solely dependent on the acquisition of motor skills and perceptual patterns but also on the structuring of the inner world of the child's mind. This is not a 'tabula rasa' but a seething mass of contradictory forces and fantasies, which he must also learn to inhibit when inappropriate. For this reason, it is not surprising that the difficulties of learning methods of communication are often associated with emotional disorders.

A speech defect is a deviation which attracts attention or affects adversely either the speaker or listener. About 10% of children have a speech defect but the incidence becomes less in later age groups. From the age of 6 to 10, 15% are affected but from 10 to 14, this decreases to 5%.

Stammering is one of the common causes of speech difficulty in childhood (see Chapter 8). Less than 10% of the speech defects are due to cerebral palsy and only 1% due to a cleft palate. Ten per cent of the defects are in the sphere of language and only 1% are due to dysphonia.

Speech disorders in children may be due to temporary or permanent interruptions in the normal ontogenetic development of speech (see pages 3 and 4). The majority of children begin to use single words when a year old but the range of normality is wide stretching from 8 months to $2\frac{1}{2}$ years. Words are put together in phrases at about 18 months, again with a wide range from 10 months to $3\frac{1}{2}$ years. In most children, speech is intelligible to the family and friends by the age of 2, but one child in three passes through a phase of unintelligible speech during the third and fourth years. Development does not take place at a steady rate; words are used and lost again and there are often silent periods when little progress is made.

The development of speech depends upon hearing and linking of the sounds and symbols of the spoken word. Poor speech development may result from disorders of 'hearing', 'language', or 'articulation' and many children have multiple disabilities.

The development of speech should be regarded as abnormally delayed if the child is not speaking by the age of $3\frac{1}{2}$ years old. If deafness can be excluded (see Chapter 7) the commonest cause of delayed development of speech is mental defect. Information regarding this can be gathered from the child's milestones, e.g.

holding head up—three months
sitting   —six months
standing   —nine months
walking   —twelve months

Other milestones include feeding himself, being clean and dry, ability to dress, playing alone and character of play.

There may be psychological or emotional causes of delayed speech, and a deprived child may not have the stimulus to speak, e.g. because of being in an institution. With all speech disorders, boys are more commonly affected than girls, and this is particularly so in stammering (see Chapter 8).

The importance of cerebral dominance is controversial in developmental speech disorders but left-handedness and ambidexterity appear commoner both in affected children and their relatives; in one series 5% of normal children were left-handed whereas 50% of the affected children showed signs of cerebral ambilaterally, i.e. mixed dominance with a combination of, say, left-handedness and right-eyedness. The failure to establish a completely dominant hemisphere is not necessarily the cause of the delayed speech but may be an associated abnormality of brain function.

CLASSIFICATION:

The diagnosis of disorders of speech and language in children can be one of inordinate complexity. Not only does it involve many disciplines but the decision as to whether speech is delayed for pathological reasons can also be difficult. These can be classified into disorders:

1. of articulation
    (a) neurological (see Chapters 10 and 11)
    (b) mechanical (e.g. hare-lip)
    (c) dyslalia
2. of voice—dysphonia (see Chapter 12)
3. of language—developmental dysphasia
4. of reading and writing—developmental dyslexia and dysgraphia
5. of rhythm—chiefly stammering (see Chapter 8)
6. secondary to
    (a) deafness—central and peripheral (see Chapter 7)
    (b) mental factors—amentia or subnormality
    (c) psychiatric factors (autism, elective mutism)
    (d) environmental factors (lack of stimulus)

Dyslalia is the immature pronunciation of words, for which there is no obvious structural cause. This may occur in isolation or be part of a more general retardation of speech and language development.

Children over the age of 5 with immature patterns of speech (e.g. speech may be like that of a three year old) may lisp, e.g. have rhoticism where there is difficulty with 'r' or sigmatism where there is difficulty with 's'. These immature forms of speech are grouped together as 'dyslalia'. There is no defect in the nervous system apart from the continuing immature speech—lips, tongue and palate move normally when tested and these is no apraxic difficulty so that there is normally a rapid response to appropriate treatment, e.g. practising the proper pronunciation of words under supervision. Dyslalia must be differentiated from articulatory dyspraxia (apraxic dysarthria) in which children are unable to imitate speech sounds, so that their response to treatment is much less satisfactory. Dyslalia must also be differentiated from the other forms of 'lalling' or idioglossia.

Disorders of Language—Developmental Dysphasia

There are many different types and several synonyms which lead to confusion. These include developmental dysphasia, congenital auditory imperception, word deafness, audimutitas, idiopathic language retardation, developmental speech disorder syndrome (Ingram, 1969).

Many of the terms suggest an aetiological cause or anatomical substrate which has not yet been proven.

The terms congenital or developmental dysphasia are paradoxical in that dysphasia—as strictly defined—is the loss of the ability to express or understand speech after it has been acquired; this differs from defects of speech which come on before speech has been fully developed. The same sort of difference exists between dementia (which is the loss or disintegration of the established mental functions) and amentia (which is the failure of developmental of mental functions).

In the case histories of children with developmental dysphasia, the condition is sometimes familial. There is often a history of birth trauma as evidenced by difficult labour, breech delivery, twin preganncy, forceps or precipitate delivery and prematurity. Babble is not well developed and this is a significant feature since other milestones may be normal. The speech disturbances may vary from mild distortions of language structure and content to severe degrees of linguistic failure. There may then be an overall retardation of language development or a specific language disorder.

There is also another group in which the dysphasia is acquired in childhood. These children develop speech normally, i.e. pre-linguistic babble is normal and, depending on the age of onset, two-word phrases and sentences are spoken. Between the ages of $2\frac{1}{2}$ and 6, during a period of days or a few weeks, hearing appears to be lost and then speech goes, perhaps with a stammer, so that within a short time these children may become completely aphasic. Epileptic attacks may occur at, or soon after, the onset. Although tumours etc. have to be exlcuded, investigations such as X-rays of the skull, cerebro-spinal fluid (C.S.F.) analysis, air encephalography and carotid arteriography are almost invariably normal. The electroencephalogram (E.E.G.) is usually abnormal especially over the temporal area on the dominant side; these E.E.G. abnormalities, like the fits, usually subside spontaneously over the ensuing few months or years.

Like adult aphasia, the speech defect may be mainly on the expressive side, i.e. these children can understand most of what is said especially if it is spoken slowly, but in the more severe cases they cannot. The failure to speak in these cases is often compensated for by gesture, and encouragement and training in the use of mime may be a valuable aid to their therapy.

Another clinical difference between the 'developmental' and

'acquired' groups is the sex incidence. The developmental cases, like those with specific dyslexia and stammerers are more commonly boys but the acquired group shows no predilection for either sex.

As would be expected, the acquired cases show psychiatric disturbances, e.g. temper-tantrums, mood changes and alteration in personality which may mistakenly suggest a psychogenic aetiology. These are not so common in the congenital group.

In developmental receptive dysphasia (congenital word deafness), there is difficulty in discriminating and appreciating the significance of the sounds heard. The diagnosis cannot be made until the age is reached at which normal children would begin to speak. It should be suspected if the child takes no notice when spoken to and does not repeat words. The diagnosis is made difficult by the variable responses to sound, e.g. these children may respond to their names at some times but not at others. Audiometry should always be done as this often shows a loss in the higher frequency ranges. This may improve over the years, but whether to conditioning or 'maturation' is uncertain. Evoked potentials with sound using E.E.G. recordings during sleep (E.E.G. audiometry) reveal responses in the auditory areas if peripheral deafness is not the primary disturbance.

Routine neurological examination of both these groups is usually negative, i.e. very rarely are 'hard' signs such as brisk reflexes or extensor plantar responses found but there is evidence of 'soft' signs of motor dysfunction if measured by the Lincoln-Osaretsky test. For this reason these children are thought to have 'minimal brain damage'.

Even in the absence of neurological signs there can be little doubt that the cause is physiogenic (i.e. organic), but it is difficult to state 'where' and 'what' the lesion is. The localisation of a lesion is not the same as the localisation of a function and attempts to understand children's speech disturbances by analogies with adult lesions may be deceptive and unjustifiable. However the anatomical site of the defect is possibly the inferior parietal lobule (supramarginal and angular gyri, Brodmann's areas 39 and 40). This is the 'association area of association areas' upon which projection fibres from the primary motor, sensory, visual and auditory areas impinge. This area is particularly important since speech depends on the ability to form cross-modal associations. The inferior parietal lobule is unique to man (as is speech) and like all recent evolutionary areas in the brain, myelinates late and also shows late dendrogenesis (formation of dendrites). It is possible to speculate that the rapidly growing and 'maturing' area is peculiarly sensitive to noxious stimuli and produces the 'disconnection syndrome' of developmental aphasia.

Developmental (specific) Dyslexia

A difference of at least two years between mental and reading ages is probably outside normal limits and the term specific or developmental dyslexia is used; because the range of normality is so wide some educationalists have doubted the existence of specific dyslexia.

The commonest cause of backwardness in reading is subnormal intelligence with diminution of the overall learning ability. In border-line cases formal assessment of the intelligence quotient by psychological testing is helpful. In some children difficulties arise because they are distractable and restless with poor attention span. This may be due to the syndrome of 'chronic minimal brain damage', which is manifest as backwardness in reading, writing, speaking or clumsy movements, often with a hyperkinetic state or other behaviour disorders. Milestones may be normal but, if delayed, can give an indication of brain damage and there may be corroborative evidence in the history. On psychological testing visuo-spatial abnormalities are often found so that there is reversal or transposition of letters at a later age than normal.

There is often an inconsistency in the mistakes, the child at one time being able to read or write a letter or word but not at another time. These children are often able to mirror-write and mirror-read. Reading and writing of letters are often much better than of words.

Other causes of difficulty in learning to read must be excluded, e.g. visual defect, poor teaching (large classes or poor school attendance) and difficulty in home circumstances. Another cause is an emotional block (said to be the cause in the difficulty in reading of Hans Christian Andersen).

The age incidence of diagnosis is between 6 and 9 years. Boys suffer from this far more commonly than girls in the proportion of 5 to 1. Hallgren gave a rough estimate of the incidence of specific dyslexia as 10%. There is often a history of twinning in the family with concordance in monozygotic twins and discordance in 2/3 of dizygotic twins. There is often a family history of dyslexia and there may be an increased incidence of left-handedness in relatives. The significance of left-handedness depends on the criteria used for testing hand dominance. The various difficulties in reading consist of:

(1) inability to work out the pronunciation of a strange word
(2) failure to see likeness and differences in forms of words
(3) failure to see differences in shapes of letters
(4) making reversals
(5) failure to keep the place
(6) failure to read from left to right
(7) poor concentration
(8) failure to read with sufficient understanding

Table 1 shows the main headings for a simple clinical assessment of speech defects in children. Tests must of course be geared to the age of the child and it should be emphasised that a complete and accurate assessment needs a multidisciplinary team which would include an educational psychologist and audiologist as well as a speech therapist.

TABLE I. Examination of developmental disorders of speech in children

A. **Receptive**
    (1) Auditory acuity
    (2) Reaction to sounds
    (3) Speech comprehension with face seen
    (4) Speech comprehension with face unseen
    (5) Comprehending pantomime

B. **Expressive**
    (1) Noises
    (2) Words
    (3) Pantomime

C. **Reading**

D. **Writing**

E. **Cerebral dominance**

F. **General behaviour**
    (1) Interaction with other people
    (2) Interaction with animals, objects, tests

The commonest difficulties found are confusion of letters which have a visual resemblance, such as 'p' and 'q', 'b' and 'd'. More often a child can read the individual letters but makes mistakes with them when reading words. The mistakes made in reading do not differ from those made by a normal child learning to read. The reading speed is reduced and, in addition, the understanding of what has been read is also reduced.

There are often associated writing disabilities, viz. confusion or disfigurement of letters, errors in linking together letters with contamination, mirror-writing, block letters and reversals.

These children may also have (1) disorders of motility, for example dyspraxia, (2) minor sensory disorders, (3) inadequate directional motions, (4) right-to-left confusion with alterations in body image and simultanagnosia, and possibly (5) a faulty estimation of time.

Aetiological explanations include:

(1) a specific lesion near the angular gyrus
(2) delayed maturation in the parieto-occipital area
(3) disturbed Gestalt function
(4) lack of cerebral dominance

CHAPTER 7
DEAFNESS

The development of normal speech is largely dependent on the ability to hear and deafness, if congenital or acquired in infancy, will delay or prevent normal speech development. In any speech disorder of childhood, it is essential to ascertain whether or not there is any hearing defect.

Hearing is the reception of sound by the ear and should be distinguished from listening which is the act of paying attention to what is heard with the object of interpreting its meaning.

The cochlear system is fully developed by twelve weeks of intrauterine life, although much of the auditory system develops after birth. Although in the new born, hearing produces reflex activity, it does not become discriminatory until about nine months of age.

There are two types of deafness; *perceptive*—where there is a lesion of the auditory nerve or inner ear, and *conductive*—when there is a disorder of the middle ear. Deafness is of the conductive type with no abnormality of the auditory nerve in about 40% of cases. Patients with conductive deafness sometimes hear better in noisy surroundings and may speak more softly; those with perceptive deafness tend to confuse speech sounds and speak louder than necessary.

A tuning fork will be heard better by bone conduction than air conduction in conductive deafness, as opposed to a normal person who will hear it better by air conduction; a patient with perceptive deafness may not hear by bone conduction at all. To be certain of the degree of deafness a quantitative test of hearing such as pure tone audiometry is necessary.

DEAFNESS IN CHILDREN

The incidence of deafness in children, viz children requiring deaf education is 1·3/1,000. From the point of view of speech development the age of onset is important. Prior to the advent of antibiotics, otitis media was the commonest cause of conductive deafness in a school

The onset of deafness in adults does not usually interfere with the ability to speak, except that some will tend to shout owing to difficulty gauging the loudness of their voice. Those with deafness due to oto-sclerosis (usually familial) tend to speak more quietly than normal. Obviously communication will become more difficult as deafness increases, although in some cases a hearing aid may help. Eventually lip-reading and sign language may be necessary. If a deaf person be-comes dysphasic the deafness will obviously add to the problems of speech therapy.

Progressive unilateral deafness in adults requires careful otological and neurological investigation, in case it is due to an acoustic neuroma. This may occasionally be associated with dysarthria due to compression of the brain stem or cerebellar hemisphere by the tumour (see pages 116 and 117).

Deafness resulting from disorders of the peripheral hearing mech-anism (i.e. the ear and auditory nerve) must be distinguished from difficulty with comprehension due to receptive dysphasia and mental defects. It is very important that there should be no confusion regard-ing terms such as word deafness, cortical deafness and auditory imperception, which describe disabilities of cerebral origin and need different consideration from the usual meaning of deafness, which implies an impairment of the acuity of hearing due to a disorder affecting the peripheral hearing mechanism.

CHAPTER 8

STAMMERING

There is a vast literature, but little agreement, on the causation of stammering. From one centre alone up to 1955 there were 153 dissertations and 255 publications, and since then the number of reports from all over the world make an analysis of the findings difficult. The main area of dispute is whether stammering is simply an expression of neurosis ('the psychogenic' theory), or whether it has an organic basis (the 'physiogenic' theory) or whether it is due to a combination of both. There is no doubt that anxiety states occur in many stammerers but whether they are primary or secondary is controversial.

Nomenclature is made difficult because of the use of other terms. Stuttering is the term more commonly used in the United States and some authorities suggest that it is a more severe form of stammering or has a different aetiological background. The two terms are here considered as synonymous.

Definition

Stammering is a deviation of speech which attracts attention or affects adversely the speaker or listener because of an interruption in the normal rhythm of speech by involuntary repetition, prolongation or arrest of sounds. This does not take into account the unreliable judgement of listener or speaker—what is stammering to one person is not necessarily so to another; one speaker may consider that he is stammering when he is not and vice versa. During the development of speech, most children repeat syllables and words (echolalia), and some normal adults stammer under emotional stress, in just the same way as habitual stammerers. In normal children between the ages of two and five years old there is a repetition of words, syllables or phrases about 45 times in every 1000 running words, the upper limit being 100 times per 1000 running words. More than this produces a noticeable stammer.

Incidence

This depends on the age of the series investigated. In children of school age estimates have varied from 0·7% to 4% whereas in adults the incidence is 0·5%. This means that there are about a quarter of a million stammerers in this country and over 15 million stammerers in the world.

Age of onset

Eighty-five per cent of those who stammer begin to do so before the age of 8; there are probably two peaks, namely at about 2–3 years, when the child starts to speak and 6–8 years when the child learns to read soon after starting school and mixing with other children; relatively few start to stammer after the age of 10 years.

Sex incidence

Like speech defects in general, it is commoner in boys; the exact proportion, like its frequency, varies with age. Stammering tends to persist more with boys so that the discrepancy of incidence in the two sexes increases with age. Under the age of 6 years there are twice as many boys as girls affected whilst at all ages there are probably seven times as many males as females affected.

Genetic factors

There is a familial incidence of stammering varying in different series from 36% to 65%. These estimates show a wide discrepancy because of the differences in defining a stammerer and the type of relatives included, e.g. whether only first degree relatives (or also cousins, uncles and grandparents as well as parents and siblings). The familial incidence does not necessarily imply a genetic factor since environmental factors could also apply to more than one member of the family and, since mimicry is one of the modes of learning in children, imitation is a powerful factor. In families with stammerers, twins are more likely to stammer than the other children. Stammering in some series, but not others, was found to be more common in identical than non-identical twins but, in these cases, the sex incidence does not show the usual male preponderance. Interestingly, the incidence of stammering is greater in families in which twinning occurs than in families without twins.

Stammering occurs more frequently with consonants than vowels in the proportion of about 5 to 1; the vast majority of stammering incidents (96%) are associated with the initial sounds of the word.

Factors that improve stammering are: (1) speaking in unison, (2) modifying the voice by singing, whispering, acting or using a different pitch, (3) repetition of rhymes, stories and choral speaking.

Aggravating factors include emotional states such as anxiety and anger (although this latter sometimes improves it), rapid speech, answering questions and speaking to superiors.

Experimentally, it has been shown that people with normal speech may have their speech disturbed by delayed playback speech, i.e. playing a tape record back through well-fitting headphones with speech delayed 1/10 to 1/5 seconds. With this there is an excessive drawling of vowels with word repetition and stammering. It may be significant that the time period necessary to produce the maximum effect with delayed auditory feedback is approximately the same as the average time period taken for a syllable, viz. 0·18–0·20 seconds. This suggests that the production of speech involves a closed-cycle feed-back by which means a speaker continually monitors and checks his own voice production. With delayed feedback, it has been found that when speech sounds are repeated voluntarily, they tend to be continued involuntarily; this can be likened to the facilitation seen in reflex behaviour. Stammering can be almost totally inhibited by interfering with a stammerer's perceptions suggesting that the determining defects are perceptual rather than motor. Auditory perception may be interfered with by deafness or by compelling transference of the speaker's perceptions to a source of sound other than his own speech. Stammering is less common in deaf children.

Shadowing, i.e. copying the speech of another person, is an imitative motor action which often abolishes stammer, presumably because the subjects perception is transferred away from his own voice to the control speaker's voice. Some stammerers have no speech difficulty when singing in a choir or reciting in unison—this is not the same as shadowing because the stimulus is learned. In simultaneous reading, the control could change the text, or even speak gibberish and yet the stammerer continues to read the original text without stammering; this suggests it is not words or the interpretation of semantic concept which exercises control over the stammerer but the sounds themselves, or some elements of the sounds, which may simply act as a distraction.

When a person hears his own voice he hears it by bone and air conduction whereas, in shadowing, he hears it only by air conduction. These pathways differ in their acoustic properties. The stimuli are comparable in loudness but there is a difference in the pitch of sounds transmitted (cf. listening to one's own recorded voice where we hear our own speaking voices at a higher pitch because bone-conducted sounds manifest a low frequency emphasis).

Reflex stammering

Within recent years considerable research has been done on the reflex mechanisms involved in speech. These involve receptors in the larynx, viz. (1) in the mucosa which alter reflexly the tone of vocal cord muscles, (2) in the muscles augmenting tone of opposing muscles, and (3) in the joints which reflexly alter the tone of laryngeal muscles.

These laryngeal reflexes are co-ordinated with the voluntary action of speech so that the laryngeal muscles are *preset* up to $\frac{1}{2}$ second before the utterance of sound produces by the expiratory air stream. A fault in the presetting mechanism could explain stammering, particularly why it is nearly always initial sounds that are affected and why stammering does not occur with recitation or singing.

Organic stammerers

Electrical stimulation of the brain can produce stammer. Stammer can develop during the course of organic brain disease and differs from habitual stammer in that the sex incidence is equal, and singing or speaking in rhythm or unison will not diminish its severity. 'Organic' stammerers, like habitual stammerers, are worse under stress and may show accompanying facial grimacing and circumlocution. Habitual stammerers have been cured by neurosurgical operations which have changed cerebral ambilaterality of speech, as evidenced by Wada's text, into a unilateral cerebral dominance (Jones, 1966).

Cerebral dominance

Estimates of sinistrality amongst stammerers vary because of differences in testing handedness and footedness etc. In one series 11% were left-handed and 5% left-sided, as opposed to 6% and 3% respectively in controls.

Earlier reports suggested that the majority of stammerers were cases of shifted sinistrality but this has not been generally confirmed.

Left-handedness is commoner in twins, 10% being sinistrals as opposed to the expected 4%. Over 5% of twins stammer which is more than five times the expected number, and it has been suggested that there was a genetic link between twinning, stammering and sinistrality. Electroencephalography in some cases shows that the alpha rhythm is more symmetrical in stammerers (normally the alpha waves are of lower voltage on the dominant side); this suggests less complete dominance but there is no statistical difference between stammerers and normals.

Imperfect lateralisation for speech indicates lack of cerebral dominance (cerebral ambilaterality) and although this does not imply any psychological abnormality the 'possessor of this type of cerebral organisation is particularly vulnerable to the effects of stress' (Zangwill, 1960). There is little doubt that cerebral dominance for speech is much stronger with right-handed people than sinistrals, i.e. bihemispheric representation of speech is commoner in the latter. In the ambilateral, the proper development of reading and writing, spatial judgement and directional control is relatively easily disturbed, e.g. by brain injury at birth, or by problems in psychological adjustment. A bilingual upbringing, for example, is often noted in stammerers and may be a significant factor in some cases.

It seems likely that stammering has a multifactorial aetiology which includes a constitutional predisposition, incomplete cerebral dominance and environmental factors.

CHAPTER 9
DYSPHASIA

History

Probably the earliest case of aphasia ever recorded is in the first chapter of the Gospel according to St. Luke, where Zacharias was struck dumb but could still write (vv 20–22, and 62–64), and the next in Roman times, when about A.D. 30 Valerius Maximus described a learned man of Athens who lost his memory for letters after being struck by a stone. There were several reports of aphasia in the seventeenth, and eighteenth centuries by Linnaeus the great botanist, Morgagni, Heberden and also Goethe in his novel 'Wilhelm Meister'.

The early descriptions explained aphasia on a motor basis in terms of paralysis of the tongue and other organs of speech ('The dead palsy'), and occasionally as part of a general loss of mental faculties (Willis, 1683). A century later, when it was observed that aphasia could occur without motor paralysis and without overall dementia, the phenomenon was classed as a defect of memory. With the influence of phrenological studies in the nineteenth century, specific cerebral lesions of the organ of language were described.

In April 1861 Dr. Paul Broca had under his care at the Bicêtre Hospital in Paris a speechless hemiplegic patient. The patient eventually died and, at post-mortem examination, a cavity the size of a hen's egg was found in the posterior third of the left second and third frontal convolutions (the equivalent of Brodmann's area 44). This was demonstrated by Broca at a meeting of the Société d'Anthropologie de Paris; and as similar cases were collected, he formed the axiom: 'on parle avec l'hémisphère gauche'. (There is controversy as to whether the priority given to Broca for his discovery is justified. Dr. Mark Dax of Montpellier, according to his son Gustave, had written a paper in 1836 to the effect that lesions interfering with speech lay in the left hemisphere. This paper was not published until 1865 and Broca did not know about it at the time of his original communication.) Broca called the speech disorder 'aphemia'; previously it had been called 'alalia'. The term aphasia, which had been used in a philosophical

46

sense in the second century A.D. by the Romans, was reintroduced by Trousseau in 1864. Following this, the concept of cerebral dominance was developed.

During the last 100 years there has been considerable debate as to the best way in which to classify the disorders of speech which result from a lesion in the dominant hemisphere, and writers on the subject have included Hughlings Jackson in this country, Charcot, Marie and Dejerine in France, and Henschen and Kleist in Germany.

As mentioned in Chapter 2, there is still controversy as to whether various parts of the cortex are solely concerned with specific functions and whether a lesion of part of the speech mechanism will produce some impairment of all other aspects. Pierre Marie in 1906 attacked all the existing theories regarding aphasia (and for this reason was described by Head as 'the iconoclast') and later in 1917, with his colleague Foix, demonstrated the anatomical extent of the speech territory from a study of brain wounds identifying five zones, lesions of which produced particular varieties of speech disorders. They concluded that pure motor aphasia ('anarthrie') was the only speech disorder that could occur in isolation. In 1926 Head reported a series of 26 cases and his work achieved great significance from the fine detail in which his patients were studied and the brilliant discussion of the problems revealed by the clinical findings. Kleist (1934) reported detailed studies of similar material from Germany but, unlike Head, he attempted to elucidate a large number of clinical syndromes, each corresponding with small areas of cortical damage. Henschen (1920, 1922) also attempted to localise separate aspects of language function with evidence from over 1300 cases in the literature.

Whereas before and during the early part of the twentieth century, most workers concentrated on localisation of speech functions and tended to ignore their setting in the hierarchy of higher cerebral function, the pendulum has swung back again to the holistic approach linking speech with memory and the other mental faculties.

The patho-physiology of aphasia is the most difficult in neurology. A word may be regarded as a sequence of auditory events (phonemes) and there is an average of 5 phonemes per word. English is normally spoken at the rate of 120 words per minute, so each phoneme lasts about 10 milliseconds (1/100th sec). Some phonemes have more significance than others and consonants provide more information than vowels (so that some languages, e.g. Hebrew, can dispense with the latter). Not every phoneme is appreciated but there is a redundancy in speech so that other factors, such as rhythm and intonation, are important.

Definition

Dysphasia may be defined as the loss of ability to formulate, express or understand the meaning of spoken words; in addition, there may be failure to understand written words (dyslexia), gestures, signs (asymbolia) or music (amusia). With dysphasia there is confusion in the expression and understanding of speech and language due to a focal cerebral lesion; it has to be distinguished from general mental confusion which results from more diffuse disorders of cerebral function. This distinction is often difficult but mental confusion includes disturbances of thought processes, intellectual ability and behaviour as well as speech and memory.

The terms aphasia (alexia etc.) strictly indicate a complete loss of function, whereas dysphasia (dyslexia etc.) imply partial loss; however the prefix a- and dys- are often used interchangeably.

Clinical types

Traditionally dysphasia is divided into expressive or executive defects (*motor dysphasia*) and receptive defects (*sensory dysphasia*). Although either expressive or receptive defects may predominate, elements of both are usually present. Speech requires the combined activity of the mechanisms of movement, hearing, and seeing and these are completely interdependent; a lesion, even a small one, that interrupts connections between them may cause catastrophic effects on all aspects of speech. This type has been called *central* or *global aphasia*.

Since speech is originally developed in relation to hearing words, auditory organisation remains the fundamental scaffolding on which all else is built. Thus damage to the auditory area and its storage systems puts most aspects of speech out of action. Speech is heard but not understood by the patient (*word deafness*) and if he talks it is unintelligible (*jargon*). Because of this patients are almost devoid of rational thought or action. Writing is usually impossible (*dysgraphia*) although the ability to copy letters may be preserved, and reading will also be lost (*dyslexia*). This global effect suggests that even if parts of the speech mechanisms are normal, they are rendered useless by damage to the central speech organisation.

Inability to name objects is called *nominal* or *amnestic* dysphasia. Patients may be unable to construct sentences (*syntactical dysphasia*) or use a jumble of meaningless words (*jargon dysphasia*). These are descriptive clinical divisions which may be associated with receptive or expressive defects. Patients with expressive dysphasia commonly realise their disability and, for this reason, are disinclined to attempt to speak. Those with receptive or sensory dysphasia commonly do not realise their mistakes and may talk excessively (*logorrhoea*). Disturbances of inflexion, stress and rhythm (*dysprosody*) are other features which may occur.

Dysphasia has also been classified in terms of fluency. Non-fluent speech with reduced word output, poor articulation and disturbed rhythm, as a form of expressive dysphasia, results from a lesion in the region of the inferior frontal convolution of the dominant cerebral hemisphere (Broca's area) or of its connections, i.e. in the anterior part of the language area. A lesion in the posterior part of the upper temporal convolution (Wernicke's area) or temporo-parietal lobe of the dominant cerebral hemisphere interferes with comprehension causing receptive (sensory) dysphasia often associated with circumlocution, neologisms and distortion of words or syllables but speech remains fluent with normal articulation and rhythm.

Dysphasia, in addition to causing difficulty in speaking, often affects the intellect as well but the patient retains *non-intellectual speech*. This consists of:

(1) *emotional utterances:* e.g. (a) ejaculations or expostulations,

   (b) 'Yes' and 'No' which are primitive words in the sense that they are among the first to be learnt,
   (c) other words used inappropriately or without regard to their proper sense,
   (d) *jargon*, where words are meaningless and unintelligible,
   (e) *recurrent utterances* of words or phrases which are sometimes those that were used just before the lesion occurred,

(2) *automatic speech:* such as songs and poems,

(3) *serial speech:* such as the alphabet, days of the week or months of the year,

(4) *social gesture speech:* such as 'How do you do' or 'Goodbye'

Some of these forms of speech may be retained by virtue of the contribution by the non-dominant hemisphere.

Expressive Dysphasia

This is similar to the 'verbal aphasia' of Head, in which there is defective formation of words and when severe, the patient may be unable to say anything. In the less severe form, or during recovery, the patient may be able to speak in a telegram style leaving out prepositions and conjunctions (*telegrammatism*), with a general poverty of spontaneous speech. There may be grammatical errors (*paragrammatism* or *syntactical aphasia*) with confusion of articles and conjunctions. Disorders of word formation, resulting in faulty pronunciation (cortical or apraxic dysarthria, also called *articulatory apraxia*) occur sometimes with reversion to spoonerisms, use of wrong words and difficulty with word finding. *Perseveration* of words is also a characteristic feature; it is the inappropriate repetition of the same reply to different questions. *Paraphasia* is the name given to disorders of sentence formation and is not to be confused with *periphrasis*, a circumlocutory way of saying things which also occurs in this type of dysphasia.

Some patients are unaware of their mistakes but those with nominal aphasia will usually recognise the correct name when it is offered. This could be due to a loss of memory for the appropriate word (amnestic aphasia). There may also be a failure to recognise the significance or intention of words or phrases (*semantic aphasia*).

Pure word dumbness is another type of expressive aphasia with loss of spontaneous speech and writing, and inability to read aloud although the patient is still able to repeat words or phrases and write by copying or on dictation. Such patients are able to tap out the number of syllables in a word (which patients with other types of expressive aphasia cannot do). A possible explanation is that there is an interruption between the cortical centre for storage of words and the motor pathways of articulation.

Receptive Aphasia

Auditory-word deafness

In auditory-word deafness, words although heard are not understood, they fail to convey their normal meaning. In a less severe form, individual words may be recognised and understood but the meaning of sentences is not appreciated. This could be classified as an agnosia for words and there may even be auditory agnosia for sounds so that a patient may be unable to interpret the significance of sounds, for example the rattle of a bunch of keys.

These types of 'deafness' are not due to any defect of the peripheral mechanism of hearing, but there is a failure to appreciate the significance or meaning of sounds transmitted to, or received by, the auditory area. If this part of the dominant hemisphere is damaged, receptive dysphasia and, when severe, auditory agnosia are likely to result. If damage is confined to the corresponding part of the non-dominant hemisphere, there may be no noticeable effect. Destruction of the auditory areas bilaterally causes cortical deafness, i.e. a complete failure to recognise any sound even though the peripheral mechanism for hearing is intact. Thus the non-dominant hemisphere contributes to the control of speech by the dominant hemisphere, the corpus callosum being the main connection between the two hemispheres. Recovery of speech after severe lesions of the dominant left hemisphere may also depend on the functioning of the right hemisphere, and an additional lesion of the *right* parietal lobe or corpus callosum will probably prevent the redevelopment of language functions.

THE EXAMINATION OF THE APHASIC PATIENT

There are many different methods of clinical and psychological assessment of aphasia (e.g. Schuell's), and most differ only in detail and the order of tests performed.

It is important to remember that a dysphasic patient fatigues more easily than a normal person and that concentration is impaired; for these reasons several interviewing periods may be necessary. For clinical purposes the following routine proves helpful.

(1) Preliminary assessment of:
   (a) general mental state, e.g. disorientation in space and time, confusion,
   (b) hearing,
   (c) vision, e.g. homonymous hemianopia or other visual field defect,
   (d) motor function, e.g. hemiparesis.

(2) Cerebral dominance: which hand, leg or eye is preferred.

(3) Receptive function:
(a) response to spoken questions and commands, initially simple and then more complex.
If incorrect response, note whether mistakes are recognised.
(b) response to written questions and commands, picking out from a group of objects the one that is written down.

(4) Expressive function:
(a) speech—spontaneity, quantity and fluency.
The correctness of word formation, sentence construction and reading.
The presence of emotional speech, the lack of propositional speech.
Singing better than speech.
Repetition of words and sentences.
Serial speech, e.g. letters of the alphabet, days of the week, months of the year, well-known sayings.
In polyglot patients ascertain which languages have been lost.
Naming objects if nominal defect; can use of objects be described.
Recognition of correct names and colours.
(b) writing—spontaneous (not only name and address, which are often 'automatic') names of objects shown, writing to dictation, copy writing,
(c) spelling.

(5) Other symbolic functions:
Reading numbers aloud.
Writing numbers to dictation.
Copying numbers, or copying numbers written as digits and numbers as words.
Copying geometric figures.
Drawing.
Calculation.
Music.

(6) Apraxia:
Use of objects, e.g. matches, comb, scissors, eating utensils.
Simple movements, e.g. putting out tongue, showing teeth, waving goodbye, dressing.
Complicated actions.

(7) Agnosia and disorders of body image:
    Distinction between right and left, getting in and out of bed,
    finding way, recognition of objects, test for finger agnosia.

CAUSES OF APHASIA

The pathological conditions which most commonly cause aphasia are:

(1) cerebral vascular disorders (see Chapter 17)
(2) intracranial tumours (see Chapter 16)
(3) cerebral abscess (see Chapter 18)
(4) brain injuries (see Chapter 19)

In fact there are many diseases which can interfere with the cerebral
control of speech and language. Aphasia is thus not a pathological
diagnosis, but merely a manifestation of any lesion of the speech area.
Occasionally it occurs as an isolated deficit, although in most cases
there are associated disturbances of cerebral function, such as a right
upper motor neurone type of facial weakness or hemiparesis. However
the aphasia and hemiparesis may develop or recover independently of
each other.

Aphasia may also occur as a transitory phenomenon in migraine or
as the aura of a focal epileptic attack.

Developmental speech and language disorders are described separately
in Chapter 6.

PROGNOSIS OF APHASIA

The degree of recovery from aphasia depends upon many factors, the
chief being the following:

1. The site and extent of the lesion, e.g. which part and how much of
   the speech area has been affected, whether the non-dominant
   hemisphere and commissures have been damaged.
2. The cause of the lesion, e.g. whether the pathological process is
   reversible or progressive, benign or malignant.
3. Treatment of the cause, response to drugs or radiotherapy, whether
   surgical removal of a tumour has been total or partial.
4. Speech therapy, stage when started.
5. The severity and clinical type of dysphasia, the more severe the

dysphasia, the greater the amount of recovery required. Severe receptive defects may make it impossible for speech therapy to be given. Associated language defects are also important, e.g. dyslexia and dysgraphia.

6. (a) Associated non-language defects, e.g. impairment of other mental functions, particularly memory, apraxia and agnosia.

(b) Other disabilities, e.g. defects of visual fields (homonymous hemianopia), ocular movements (diplopia), motor functions (hemiplegia), sensory functions (hemianaesthesia), epilepsy, dizziness.

7. (a) Psychological factors, e.g. inability to concentrate, to co-operate and to adjust to limitations, depression, emotional lability.

(b) Environmental factors, e.g. home and social conditions, help from relatives, encouragement and reassurance.

8. Age, the older the patient, the poorer the prognosis.

9. Cerebral dominance, see Chapter 5.

10. Premorbid language and intellectual ability, personality and temperament.

CHAPTER 10
DYSARTHRIA I

Dysarthria literally means disordered articulation and therefore could be due to local non-neurological causes such as cleft palate and loose fitting dentures. The term is perhaps better restricted to faulty pronunciation due to neuromuscular disorders.

The correct pronunciation of words (articulation) is dependent upon complex processes which control and co-ordinate the neuro-muscular system. The sounds recognised as words are produced by the vibration of the vocal cords in the larynx, caused by an outflow of air coming from the lungs; any interference with this mechanism produces weakness or hoarseness of the voice, dysphonia (see Chapter 12). The sounds are then given their correct form by movements of lips, tongue and palate and any abnormality of this system produces defects or difficulty in articulation, hypo- or hyper-nasality or changes in intonation.

NEUROLOGICAL CAUSES OF DYSARTHRIA

The neurological causes of dysarthria are classified according to which part of the neuromuscular system is affected. The disorders may thus involve:

(1) muscles
(2) lower motor neurones
(3) upper motor neurones
(4) extra-pyramidal system
(5) cerebellum and its connections
(6) cerebral cortex (motor speech area)

and will be described under these headings.

DISORDERS OF MUSCLES

All our active movements such as breathing, performing manoeuvres with the hands and walking, are dependent upon the action of muscles.

Likewise the muscles concerned with articulation are essential for the production of normal speech. Muscles form 80% of the body weight and there are over 200 named ones in the body. Each muscle consists of bundles of microscopic muscle fibres which are capable of contracting and relaxing under nervous control mediated by biochemical means. By virtue of the attachments of muscles, shortening of the fibres resulting from their contraction produces movement. Individual muscles are supplied by the cranial or spinal nerves which form the necessary connections with the brain stem or spinal cord respectively.

Primary disorders of muscles are referred to as 'myopathies'. They are characterised by weakness and wasting of the muscles affected with reduction or loss of associated tendon reflexes. The electrical reactions of the muscle tested by electromyography (E.M.G.) are abnormal.

The different diseases have a predilection for certain groups of muscles and can be recognised by the particular pattern and distribution of the muscles affected. Whether speech is involved will depend upon the type and extent of the disease. The main diseases that have to be considered are:

(1) the muscular dystrophies
(2) polymyositis
(3) myasthenia gravis

The chief characteristics of these diseases are indicated in Table 3.

Myasthenia gravis is due to a biochemical disorder at the neuro-muscular junction. The contraction of muscles is normally dependent on the action of acetylcholine, the substance liberated at the motor end plate when an electrical discharge reaches the nerve ending. In myasthenia gravis there is a defect of synthesis or storage of acetyl-choline, which is inhibited by the naturally occurring enzyme, cholinesterase. As a result of this, the muscles fatigue sooner than normal and become progressively weaker as they are used, but power usually recovers after a period of rest.

The condition may occur at any age but usually between 20 and 50 years; it is slightly more frequent in females. The commonest mode of presentation in about 80% of cases is with ocular symptoms such as double vision (diplopia) and drooping of the upper eyelid (ptosis). Not infrequently the voice becomes fainter (dysphonic) after talking for some time, speech may become slurred and indistinct (dysarthric) and there may be difficulty in swallowing (dysphagia). The muscles of mastication (chewing) may be affected and the jaw may become so

TABLE 3. Disorders of muscles (myopathies)

	Pathology and aetiology	Signs and symptoms		Treatment
		General	Speech	
1. Muscular dystrophies	Various types affecting different groups of muscles. Abnormalities of muscle enzymes, usually hereditary.	Weakness and wasting of affected muscles. Slow progression.	Slurred speech if articulatory muscles involved.	Nil specific.
2. Polymyositis	Inflammatory disease of muscles and sometimes skin (dermatomyositis). Usually a collagen disease, 10% associated with cancer.	Usually proximal muscles weak, painful and tender.	May be slurred and slow.	Steroids.
3. Myasthenia gravis	Biochemical disorder of neuromuscular transmission. Excessive fatiguability of muscles. 10–15% associated with tumour of thymus (thymoma).	Usually affects eye muscles causing diplopia and ptosis. Dysphagia and generalised weakness may occur.	Articulation becomes increasingly indistinct (dysarthria) and the voice weak (dysphonia). Recovery following rest or injection of tensilon or prostigmine.	Prostigmine. Thymectomy. Steroids.

weak that it has to be supported by hand. The symptoms, worse in the evenings and after using the affected muscles, are relieved by rest.

The diagnosis is usually established by giving a test dose of edrophonium (tensilon) intravenously. Within a few seconds this blocks the activity of cholinesterase; acetylcholine is then not destroyed so quickly and muscle power is restored temporarily. This relief lasts for a few minutes only and weakness then returns. Alternatively neostigmine (prostigmine) can be given intramuscularly; it has the same effect after about 15 minutes and acts for about an hour. In most cases treatment with neostigmine tablets taken by mouth is effective.

DISORDERS OF LOWER MOTOR NEURONES

The nervous impulses which control movement are transmitted along the motor pathway extending from the cerebral cortex to the peripheral nerves supplying the muscles (see Fig. 3). The parts extending from the motor nuclei of the cranial nerves along their nerve fibres to the neuro-muscular junction (the motor end plate) and from the anterior horn cells in the spinal cord along the fibres of the spinal nerves to their motor end plates constitute the *lower motor neurones* (L.M.N.).

Each nerve fibre supplies a large number of muscle fibres, the number varying with the type of muscles, e.g. the average limb muscle will have about one nerve fibre supplying 100 muscle fibres, whereas in the external ocular muscles the ratio is approximately 1 to 4. The nerve fibre together with the muscle fibres it supplies is called a 'motor unit'. The nerve cells of the lower motor neurones (i.e. the motor nuclei of the cranial nerves and the anterior horn cells of the spinal cord) are controlled by other parts of the nervous system. Thus the initiation and coordination of muscular action, and the control of tone and posture are the result of impulses from the motor nerve cells in the cerebral cortex (the upper motor neurones) interacting with impulses from the cerebellum and basal ganglia and being transmitted across the synapses to the lower motor neurones (see Fig. 5).

Synapse

A synpase is the gap between the termination of one nerve fibre and the cell body of another neurone, around which there is an area of electrical excitability highly sensitive to the chemical substances responsible for the transmission and modification of impulses.

FIGURE 5. Diagrammatic representation of control of muscle.

Disorders of the lower motor neurones are characterised by wasting
and weakness of the muscles affected, their tone is decreased leading
to flaccidity, and their tendon reflexes are reduced or absent (see Table
5). Electrical studies of nerve conduction and of the affected muscles
by electromyography (E.M.G.) show characteristic changes.

In some cases of lower motor neurone involvement, particularly
when there is active degeneration of the anterior horn cells, the affected
muscles show spontaneous small contractions—fasciculation. This can
also be shown on the electromyogram and is a typical feature of motor
neurone disease (see pages 62, 68 and 71).

The lower motor neurones controlling the muscles used for articulation (as well as phonation and swallowing) form the 7th, 9th, 10th, 11th and 12th cranial nerves originating from their motor nuclei in the brain stem. These supply the muscles of the lips, palate, pharynx, larynx and tongue, and knowledge of their anatomy is required.

Seventh cranial (facial) nerve leaves the lower border of the pons on each side and passes through the skull in the facial canal in close proximity to the eighth cranial (acoustic) nerve. It emerges through the stylomastoid foramen and supplies the muscles which control facial expression, movements of the lips, raising the eyebrows, frowning and closing the eyes.

The 9th, 10th and 11th cranial nerves leave the medulla on each side and pass through the skull in the jugular foramen.

Ninth cranial (glossopharyngeal) nerve supplies only one muscle, the stylo-pharyngeus and conveys sensation from the pharynx and posterior third of the tongue including taste.

Tenth cranial (vagus) nerve is formed by several roots emerging from the medulla oblongata. They join to form the intracranial trunk of the vagus nerve which on each side passes through the skull in the jugular foramen. Here the nerve enlarges (ganglion jugulare) to connect with the 7th, 9th 11th and 12th cranial nerves and sympathetic fibres. After passing through the jugular foramen, the vagus forms another ganglion (ganglion nodosa) which connects with sensory and parasympathetic fibres. Inferior to this ganglion, the pharyngeal plexus is formed by the pharyngeal branches of the vagus, the pharyngeal branches of the glossopharyngeal and sympathetic fibres. It is this plexus which innervates the palate and pharynx both sensory and motor, supplying (a) the muscles of the palate (with the exception of the tensor palati which is supplied by the mandibular branch of the 5th nerve) and (b) the muscles of the pharynx, namely the three constrictors, and the salpingo- and palato-pharyngeus, and the stylo-pharyngeus muscle (see above).

Next to arise from the vagus, below the pharyngeal plexus, is the superior laryngeal nerve. This divides into the internal branch conveying sensation from the laryngeal mucosa above the vocal cords, and the external branch which innervates the cricothyroid muscle. The remaining intrinsic muscles of the larynx are supplied by the recurrent laryngeal nerves which also arise from the vagus but then take a different course on the two sides, on the left curving below the arch of the aorta, and on the right below the subclavian artery. The vagus then

TABLE 4a. Disorders of lower motor neurones, involving cranial nerves 7th, 9th, 10th, 11th, 12th

	Pathology and aetiology	Signs and symptoms		Treatment
		General	Speech	
1. Polyneuritis	Acute type following infections, occasionally glandular fever etc. Chronic cases, e.g. due to diabetes and alcohol.	Symmetrcial weakness and sensory changes usually starting in distal parts of limbs and 'muzzle' area of face. Spinal and cranial nerves may be affected.	Dysarthria, nasal voice and dysphonia result if the lower cranial nerves are affected due to paresis of lips, palate, pharynx, larynx and tongue.	Rest in acute stage, postural drainage or tracheostomy and assisted respiration may be necessary.
2. Damage to cranial nerves	Neoplasm Goitre Aneurysm of aorta Trauma.	Local effects dependent on the type and site of the pathological lesion.	As above.	Sometimes surgical.
3. Bell's palsy	Inflammatory or ischaemic lesion of 7th cranial (facial) nerve in stylomastoid canal. Usually recovers.	Paralysis of the facial muscles on the affected side.	Slurred speech due to unilateral facial weakness affecting muscles around the mouth.	Physiotherapy for facial muscles. Occasionally steroids or surgery.

TABLE 4b. Disorders of lower motor neurones,
involving motor nuclei of brain stem

| | Pathology and aetiology | Signs and symptoms | | Treatment |
		General	Speech	
1. Poliomyelitis	Virus infection of motor nuclei of cranial nerves in brain stem and anterior horn cells of spinal cord. Mild cases are reversible, severe irreversible (see pages 132 and 133).	Paresis or paralysis of limb muscles with wasting and L.M.N. signs. No sensory loss. Bulbar palsy. Respiratory paralysis.	Dysarthria. Dysphonia.	As for polyneuritis.
2. Motor neurone disease	Cause unknown. Onset usually in middle age. Progressive deterioration with death usually in 2–4 years.	Progressive bulbar palsy. Wasting and fasciculation of tongue, and muscles of limbs (amyotrophy). Saliva in excess due to pharyngeal weakness with dysphagia. U.M.N.s also involved (see Table 6).	Dysarthria, articulation becomes more indistinct, labials most noticeably affected due to paresis of lips, progressive weakness of tongue impairs dental and velar sounds. Dysphonia, weakness of soft palate causes nasal tone.	Nil specific.

3. Syringobulbia (Syringomyelia)	Cystic degeneration starting around 4th ventricle and central canal of spinal cord. Developmental disorder. Onset of symptoms usually between 20 and 40. Slowly progressive.	Nystagmus. Sensory loss on face associated with manifestations of syringomyelia—i.e. wasting of small muscles of the hands, trophic changes etc.	As above.	Surgical decompression occasionally indicated.
4. Neoplasm	Glioma—rare in brain stem, usually children.	Signs of progressive involvement of cranial nerve nuclei, often starting in the pons, may be asymmetrical.	As above.	Radiotherapy.

descends through the thorax forming cardiac and gastric plexuses and supplying motor, secretory and sensory fibres to the various viscera.

Eleventh cranial (accessory) nerve is a purely motor nerve, composed of two parts, cranial and spinal. The *cranial part* joins the vagus nerve and contributes to the functions described above. The *spinal part* arises from grey matter in the lateral part of the anterior horn of the upper 5 cervical cord segments, and forms a trunk which passes upwards through the foramen magnum; it briefly makes contact with the cranial part of the accessory nerve and the vagus, and with them passes out of the skull again through the jugular foramen. It then supplies the sterno-mastoid and trapezius muscles.

Twelfth cranial (hypoglossal) nerve leaves the lower part of the medulla on each side and passes through the skull in the hypoglossal foramen. It traverses the deep structures of the neck and supplies the muscles of the tongue.

Disorders of lower motor neurones causing dysarthria are divided into two groups, depending on whether there is involvement of the cranial nerves (7th, 9th, 10th, 11th or 12th) or of their motor nuclei in the brain stem.

A. *Disorders of cranial nerves* (7, 9, 10, 11 and 12)

(1) Polyneuritis
(2) Damage by neoplasm, goitre, aneurysm or trauma
(3) Bell's palsy

B. *Disorders of motor nuclei in the brain stem*

(1) Polyiomyelitis
(2) Motor neurone disease (progressive bulbar palsy)
(3) Syringobulbia
(4) Neoplasm

For further details of these conditions, see Tables 4*a* and 4*b*. Dysarthria due to the disorders of the lower motor neurones may form part of the clinical syndrome of bulbar palsy.

BULBAR PALSY

Mechanism of production

Bulbar palsy implies that there is weakness of the muscles supplied by the cranial nerves whose motor nuclei lie in the medulla or bulb. The diseases causing bulbar palsy involve either these motor nuclei, the cranial nerves themselves, their motor end plates or the muscles supplied (see Tables 3, 4a and 4b).

Clinical features

The main clinical features are dysarthria, dysphagia and dysphonia with weakness and wasting of the muscles supplied by the lower cranial nerves. Weakness of elevation of the soft palate may fail to close off the nasopharynx, so that when speaking there is excessive nasality of the voice (hyper-rhinolalia) and when swallowing nasal regurgitation may occur particularly with fluids. In the progressive bulbar palsy due to motor neurone disease, fasciculation in the tongue and other muscles is a characteristic feature.

The dysarthria of bulbar palsy in which the weakness of the muscles is associated with wasting usually affects all consonants and differs from that of pseudo-bulbar palsy in which the muscle weakness is associated with spasticity.

Associated signs

There may be more generalised lower motor neurone involvement affecting the muscles of the trunk and limbs, supplied by the spinal nerves originating from the affected anterior horn cells of the spinal cord. These muscles will then also develop weakness, wasting and flaccidity with diminution or absence of tendon reflexes.

DISORDERS OF UPPER MOTOR NEURONES

Disorders may affect any part of the upper motor neurone from its origin in the motor cortex to its termination in the synapse with its appropriate lower motor neurone (Fig. 3). The muscles affected become weak or paralysed with no wasting or just a little due to disuse. The tone of the affected muscles is increased, leading to spasticity which is usually accompanied by the phenomenon of clonus. Clonus is typically elicited by the stimulus of stretching a muscle or group of muscles and consists of the repetitive alternating contraction and relaxation of these muscles. The clonus in severe cases is sustained as long as the stretch stimulus is applied, and can occur spontaneously. The tendon reflexes on the affected side are exaggerated and the plantar response becomes extensor (Babinski's sign). Paralysis may involve one limb (monoplegia), one half of the body (hemiplegia), both legs (paraplegia) or all four limbs (quadriplegia), depending on which of the upper motor neurone fibres are involved.

The main differences between the clinical signs of upper and lower motor neurone lesions are summarised in Table 5.

TABLE 5. Summary of the differences between upper and lower motor neurone lesions

	U.M.N.	L.M.N.
Distribution of weakness	Whole limb or part	Single muscles or groups of muscles
Tone	Increased (spasticity)	Decreased (flaccidity)
Clonus	Present	Absent
Tendon reflexes	Increased	Decreased or absent
Plantar response	Extensor	Flexor or absent
Wasting	Absent	Present
Fasciculation	Absent	Present in some

Most of the motor nuclei of the cranial nerves in the brain stem have bilateral U.M.N. representation. This means that each of these motor nuclei is controlled (1) by cortico-bulbar fibres which have originated from the contralateral cerebral hemisphere and crossed in the brain stem, i.e. the majority, and (2) by a smaller number of uncrossed cortico-bulbar fibres which have originated from the ipsilateral cerebral hemisphere. Thus cortico-bulbar fibres from both cerebral hemispheres (the majority crossed but some uncrossed) form synapses with the motor nuclei on each side of the brain stem. Part of the motor nucleus of the facial nerve supplying the muscles of the *lower* part of the face does not have bilateral representation, i.e. it is controlled only by the crossed cortico-bulbar fibres originating from the face area of the opposite cerebral hemisphere. If these upper motor neurones are damaged, there will be weakness of the muscles in the lower part of the face on the opposite side; this is in contrast to the *upper* part of the face in which power of the muscles is largely maintained because they are controlled by a different part of the nucleus of the facial nerve which does have bilateral representation, function being preserved by the uncrossed fibres originating from the unaffected cerebral hemisphere. In these cases the weakness of the face is more obvious with emotional movements than with voluntary movements of the facial muscles.

The motor nuclei of the other cranial nerves all have bilateral U.M.N. representation, and it is only the part of the motor nucleus of the facial nerve which supplies the muscles of the lower part of the face that has unilateral representation.

A tumour or haemorrhage damaging the upper motor neurones in one cerebral hemisphere produces paralysis on the opposite side of the body. This will principally affect the lower part of the face, arm and leg, producing the upper motor neurone signs mentioned, movements of the muscles which have bilateral representation being unaffected (i.e. movements of the eyes, jaws, upper part of the face, soft palate, neck and tongue).

Dysarthria only results from unilateral upper motor neurone involvement if this causes severe weakness of the facial muscles which control the lips on the affected side. Otherwise disorders of upper motor neurones must be *bilateral* to result in dysarthria, and the causes can be classified as follows:

(1) cerebral vascular lesions
(2) motor neurone disease
(3) congenital disorders—e.g. 'spastics'
(4) neoplasms—e.g. metastases
(5) miscellaneous—encephalitis, degenerative diseases, severe brain injuries

For further details of these conditions, see Table 6.

Dysarthria due to the disorders of upper motor neurones bilaterally may form part of the clinical syndrome of pseudo-bulbar palsy.

TABLE 6. Disorders of upper motor neurones (BILATERALLY) causing pseudobulbar palsy

	Pathology and aetiology	Signs and symptoms — General	Speech	Treatment
1. Cerebral vascular lesions	Arteriosclerosis. Infarction. Haemorrhage. Often associated with hypertension and heart diseases (see Chapter 17).	Often double hemi-plegia. Mental con-dition impaired. Emotional lability. Jaw jerk increased. Spasticity of face. Dysphagia. All may improve.	Slurred indistinct articulation. Voice weak (Dysphasia as well if dominant cerebral hemisphere is affected).	Nursing care during acute stages.
2. Motor neurone disease	Cause unknown. Onset usually in middle age. Progressive deterioration with death usually in 2–4 years.	Spastic weakness of muscles, including face, pharynx and limbs. Jaw jerk and limb reflexes exag-gerated. Dysphagia. Difficulty coughing. Respiratory distress. L.M.Ns also involved (see Table 4b).	Spastic type of dysarthria and dysphonia.	Nil specific.

3. Congenital disorders	Environmental and genetic causes. Cerebral palsy (see Chapter 13).	Spastic weakness of limbs, sometimes with 'scissors gait'. Mental retardation and epilepsy often but not invariably associated.	Dysarthria, may be staccato or explosive. Tongue spastic. Specific language defects.	Muscular education with relaxation exercises and physiotherapy. Speech therapy and special schooling important.
4. Neoplasms	Metastases in both cerebral hemispheres, most commonly from primary malignant tumour in lung (see Chapter 16).	Dependent on localisation of deposits. Raised intra-cranial pressure, i.e. headache, vomiting and papilloedema.	Dysarthria (may be dysphasia as well).	Radiotherapy in selected cases.
5. Miscellaneous	Encephalitis. Degenerative diseases. Severe brain injuries.	Mental confusion. Spasticity in limbs. Epilepsy.	Dysarthria. Dysphonia.	Nursing care, sometimes steroids. Speech therapy and physiotherapy, in suitable cases.

PSEUDOBULBAR PALSY

Mechanism of production

Pseudobulbar palsy is not primarily a disease of the bulb but of the cortico-bulbar fibres, i.e. that part of the upper motor neurone extending from the Betz cells in the motor cortex and terminating in the brain stem at the synpases with the motor nuclei of the cranial nerves.

The term supra-bulbar palsy is sometimes used synonymously with pseudobulbar palsy; it is accurate because it implies that the fibres above the bulb are affected and that the lesion is not actually in the bulb. The term pseudobulbar palsy is preferred because it describes the clinical state which resembles bulbar palsy.

The involvement of cortico-bulbar fibres must be *bilateral* to produce pseudobulbar palsy. This is because not all the cortico-bulbar fibres cross in the brain stem; some remain uncrossed and continue down on the same side. If the upper motor neurone lesion is unilateral the muscles supplied by the lower cranial nerves are not obviously affected (apart from the lower part of the face) and pseudobulbar palsy will not result.

Clinical features

Dysarthria and dysphagia are the main clinical effects of pseudo-bulbar palsy. The tone and reflexes of the affected muscles are increased, so there is a brisk jaw jerk, spasticity of the face and exaggeration of the palatal and pharyngeal reflexes. Spasticity in the tongue makes it appear smaller.

Associated signs

In addition to the bilateral involvement of cortico-bulbar fibres, the same diseases may affect cortico-spinal fibres producing upper motor neurone signs in the trunk and limbs with weakness, spasticity (increased tone) and clonus, exaggerated tendon reflexes and extensor plantar responses. There may be impairment of voluntary control of emotional expression, and exaggeration or prolongation of normal responses, perhaps laughing and crying for no apparent reason, causing considerable distress and embarrassment.

Causes of pseudobulbar palsy

The commonest cause of pseudobulbar palsy is *cerebro-vascular disease* involving both cerebral hemispheres. Typically there is a history of a stroke, i.e. infarction or haemorrhage in one cerebral hemisphere (see Chapter 17) followed by recovery and later a second stroke affecting the other cerebral hemisphere. The cortico-bulbar fibres may have been damaged on the side of the first stroke, but without overt signs because of the bilateral representation. Whether or not there is a residual hemiplegia, the defect of the cortico-bulbar fibres will not be apparent until the second stroke involves the opposite cerebral hemisphere whereupon pseudo-bulbar palsy results.

Motor neurone disease can also cause pseudobulbar palsy by progressive involvement of cortico-bulbar fibres bilaterally. In addition this disease may involve the cortico-spinal tracts, as well as the motor nuclei of the cranial nerves and the anterior horn cells more or less symmetrically. Thus in some cases, there will be combined features of both bulbar and pseudobulbar palsy, as well as amyotrophy and upper motor neurone signs in the limbs.

Pseudobulbar palsy may also result from *birth trauma* and *congenital defects* involving the cortico-bulbar fibres. If cortico-spinal fibres are also involved, then the pseudobulbar palsy is associated with spasticity of the limbs.

There are other causes of pseudobulbar palsy, such as bilateral *tumours of the brain* (see Chapter 16), e.g. secondary deposits (metastases) in both cerebral hemispheres.

Various combinations of these conditions can cause pseudobulbar palsy; for example a patient may have a tumour in one cerebral hemisphere, and a stroke affecting the other; one hemisphere may be damaged by a head injury, and the other by a vascular lesion or tumour. Pseudobulbar palsy results *only* from *bilateral* lesions of the cortico-bulbar pathways and the signs are those of upper motor neurone involvement.

CHAPTER 11
DYSARTHRIA 2

DISORDERS OF THE EXTRAPYRAMIDAL SYSTEM

The basal ganglia

These are nuclei of grey matter lying deep in the substance of each cerebral hemisphere. They include the globus pallidus, putamen and caudate nuclei (these three structures constitute the corpus striatum), substantia nigra, subthalamic nucleus (corpus Luysii) and the red nucleus in the upper part of the midbrain. The basal ganglia are the nuclei of the extra-pyramidal system. Via connections with other parts of the central nervous system (see Fig. 5), they help to control movement, tone and posture. The mechanism of control is complicated, but diseases of the extra-pyramidal system result in involuntary movements and disorders of tone and posture. Involuntary movements include tremor as seen in Parkinson's disease, chorea, athetosis and nallismus.

The disorders of extra-pyramidal system which can cause dysarthria are:

(1) Parkinson's disease
(2) chorea—Sydenham's (rheumatic)
    —Huntington's
(3) congenital choreo-athetosis
(4) Wilson's disease (hepato-lenticular degeneration)

The *tremor of Parkinsonism* is typically coarse and rhythmical, more marked at rest than on action. It usually starts in one hand and is classically described as 'pill-rolling'. There may be poverty of movement (hypokinesia) as well as slowness and stiffness of movements which cause a mask-like expression of the face, and rigidity of cogwheel type in the limbs. There are usually defects of fine and associated movements. The posture is often stooped and the limbs slightly flexed, the legs shuffling along so that the gait appears hurried or festinant with 'marche à petits pas'. There is no wasting, the reflexes are unaffected and the plantar responses flexor.

The speech in Parkinsonism is characteristically monotonous. Rigidity of the muscles of the larynx makes the voice weak and feeble, i.e. dysphonic. Involvement of the muscles used for articulation results in dysarthria. Speech may also be affected in a way comparable to the festinant gait, i.e. words following each other faster and faster, and the same phrase may be repeated over and over again (palilalia). In some patients, excessive salivation or difficulty in swallowing causes dribbling and slobbering which may be exaggerated by tremor of the mouth and tongue.

Chorea usually affects the peripheral parts of the limbs and causes jerky movements whilst the movements of *athetosis* are writhing, and both are purposeless and involuntary.

A lesion of the subthalamic nucleus on one side results in *hemi-ballismus* affecting the limbs on the other side of the body. Ballismic movements are involuntary, throwing, purposeless movements, affecting particularly the proximal parts of the limbs, often flinging the limb around violently.

Chorea and athetosis cause jerkiness of speech, sometimes with an explosive dysarthria due to sudden involuntary movements affecting respiratory muscles, larynx or mouth, and in severe cases speech is unintelligible.

Further details of the diseases of the extra-pyramidal system are given in Table 7.

DISORDERS OF THE CEREBELLUM

The cerebellum consists of right and left cerebellar hemispheres joined in the midline by the vermis. Each cerebellar hemisphere is connected to the corresponding side of the brain stem by three cerebellar peduncles: (1) superior (brachium conjunctivum), (2) middle (brachium pontis) and (3) inferior (restiform body).

The cerebellum and its connections control the co-ordination of movements and influence muscle tone. There are important connections with the vestibular mechanisms and cranial nerve nuclei in the brain stem concerned with movements of the muscles of the eyes and neck. The maintenance of balance and co-ordination of movements are thus dependent upon the integrity of the cerebellum and its connections.

Disturbances of cerebellar function will result in defects of co-

TABLE 7. Disorders of the extra-pyramidal system

Disease	Pathology and aetiology	Signs and symptoms General	Speech	Treatment
1. Parkinsonism	(a) Idiopathic—paralysis agitans. (b) Post-encephalitic. (c) Arteriosclerotic. (d) Toxic: 1. carbon monoxide 2. manganese 3. anoxia 4. phenothiazine drugs, e.g. chlorpromazine (largactil).	Cogwheel rigidity. Tremor, 'pill-rolling' movement of the hands. Shuffling, festinant gait. Expressionless face. Excessive salivation, drooling.	Slow with thin, feeble, monotonous voice. Dysphonia. Dysarthria. Rapid repetitions (palilalia).	Drugs, e.g. benhexol and L-dopa. Neurosurgery, e.g. stereotactic thalamotomy.
2. Chorea	(a) Sydenham's chorea, may be associated with rheumatic fever.	Choreiform movements. Grimacing, fidgeting and dropping things. Other manifestations of rheumatic fever.	Speech hesitant and jerky. Dysarthria due to jerky movements of articulatory and respiratory muscles.	Rest. Sedation. Salicylates.
	(b) Huntington's chorea. Age of onset 30–50 years. Familial. Progressive and fatal.	Choreiform movements. Dementia.	Dysarthria becoming unintelligible.	No specific treatment. Tetrabenazine.

3. **Athetosis.** (choreo athetosis)	(a) Agenesis or dysgenesis (b) Anoxia at birth (c) Severe neo-natal jaundice—'kernicterus'.	Writhing, purposeless, involuntary movements.	Explosive and indistinct. Tongue lacks voluntary control and is overactive. Facial grimacing with continual movements of lips. Irregular spasmodic contractions of diaphragm and other respiratory muscles giving jerky quality to voice.	Motor re-education with special schooling.
4. **Hepato-lenticular degeneration.** (Wilson's disease)	Familial, age of onset 10–26 years. Deficiency of copper-binding protein, caeruloplasmin, leading to deposition of copper in corpus striatum and liver.	Muscular rigidity and involuntary movements. Cirrhosis of liver causing jaundice. Deposition of copper in the cornea of the eye forming Kayser-Fleischer ring.	Rigidity of muscles affecting articulation and phonation.	Chelating agents, e.g. penicillamine.

ordination and balance, and affect speech muscles as well as the muscles of the eyes, neck, trunk and limbs.

CEREBELLAR SIGNS

Defects of one cerebellar hemisphere will cause inco-ordination in the muscles on the same side of the body (see Fig. 5). Bilateral cerebellar involvement causes generalised inco-ordination of all limbs, and lesions confined to the vermis affect co-ordination of the trunk and neck muscles.

Inco-ordination affecting the upper limbs is seen as 'intention tremor', i.e. tremor on movement; other signs include difficulty performing rapid repetitive or alternating movements (dysdiadoko-kinesis), poor control of the range of movements (dysmetria) and clumsiness. Clinical tests used to demonstrate these defects include maintenance of posture of outstretched hands and finger-nose-finger test.

Inco-ordination affects balance and causes unsteadiness when walking (ataxia) so that the patient may veer to one side and tends to sway or stumble. The maintenance of posture and control of movements of the muscles of the neck may be affected so that the head appears to jerk or waver irregularly (titubation).

Since co-ordination of eye movements is dependent upon the connections between the oculo-motor, vestibular and cerebellar pathways, cerebellar lesions are often associated with nystagmus, i.e. a rhythmical involuntary jerking movement of the eyes, usually elicited by asking the patient to look to one side, but sometimes occurring spontaneously when looking straight ahead.

The muscles of articulation may also be affected by cerebellar inco-ordination, resulting in ataxic dysarthria. In mild forms, this begins as slurring of speech and the pronunciation of consonants is particularly difficult. Speech becomes slow and thick 'as if there is something in the mouth' and slurring and jerkiness may be combined. Due to poor control of rhythm, there is a tendency to pronounce each syllable as if it is a separate word (scanning speech) and to put the emphasis on the wrong syllables, some being pronounced too loudly and others too softly (staccato speech). In severe cases speech may become explosive and unintelligible, eventually with complete inability to articulate (anarthria).

TABLE 8. Disorders of the cerebellum

Diesease	Pathology and aetiology	Signs and symptoms General	Speech	Treatment
1. Multiple sclerosis	Plaques of demyelination scattered throughout the C.N.S. and optic nerves. Irregular course of relapses and remissions. Onset 20–45 years. Females more commonly than males.	Optic neuritis. Diplopia. Vertigo. Cerebellar signs: Intention tremor Nystagmus Ataxia. Sensory disturbances. U.M.N. (pyramidal) signs.	Slurred. Scanning. Staccato. Dysphasia very rare.	Avoidance of fatigue. A.C.T.H. for acute relapses. Physiotherapy.
2. Hereditary ataxias	Friedreich's disease is the commonest affecting cerebellum, cerebellar connections, pyramidal tracts and posterior columns. Associated skeletal deformities (pes cavus, kyphoscoliosis) and cardiac abnormalities. Onset in adolescence, slowly progressive.	Cerebellar signs; U.M.N. (pyramidal) signs; posterior column signs; loss of position and vibration sense. Ataxia predominates due to cerebellar inco-ordination and loss of position sense: absent knee jerks and ankle jerks with bilateral extensor plantar responses.	Slow. Slurred. Explosive.	Aids for co-ordination. Physiotherapy, balancing exercises.

TABLE 8. Disorders of the cerebellum—*continued*

Disease	Pathology and aetiology	Signs and symptoms		Treatment
		General	Speech	
3. Degenerations	(a) Idiopathic, cerebellar atrophy. Onset later in life after 40 or 50. Slowly progressive course. No associated skeletal or cardiac disorders.	As above.	As above.	As above.
	(b) Carcinomatous degeneration usually associated with carcinoma of the bronchus. Not due to metastases in the cerebellum.	Ataxia. Cough, shadow on chest X-ray (sometimes neuropathy as well).	Dysarthria.	Nil specific. Removal of primary growth if operable, or radiotherapy.
4. Metabolic and toxic disorders	Hypothyroidism. Alcoholism.	Myxoedema. Liver disease. Bilateral cerebellar signs.	Husky voice. Dysarthria.	Thyroxine tablets. Avoidance of alcohol. Vitamin B1.

5. Congenital disorders	Agenesis or dysgenesis of cerebellum.	Oro-facial muscles under-developed. Grimacing and drooling. Lack of control of voluntary movement and of posture.	Delayed development. Slurred, jerky.	Aids for co-ordination. Physiotherapy, balancing exercises. Speech therapy.
6. Miscellaneous	(a) Vascular lesions, infarction, haemorrhage, often with hypertension.	Mainly ipsilateral cerebellar signs, sudden onset.	Dysarthria.	Operation for removal of intra-cerebellar haematoma. Nursing care. Speech therapy and physiotherapy during recovery.
	(b) Abscess, usually from otitis media (see Chapter 18). (c) Neoplasms (see Chapter 16).	Ipsilateral cerebellar signs, progressive. Raised intracranial pressure.	Dysarthria.	Antibiotics. Neurosurgery. Speech therapy and physiotherapy following operation on abscess or benign tumour.

DISEASES OF THE CEREBELLUM

(1) Multiple (disseminated) sclerosis
(2) Hereditary ataxias, e.g. Friedreich's
(3) Degenerations, e.g. idiopathic, carcinomatous
(4) Metabolic and toxic disorders, e.g. hypothyroidism, drugs (alcohol etc.)
(5) Congenital disorders, e.g. dysgenesis
(6) Miscellaneous, e.g. vascular lesions, abscess, neoplasms

Multiple Sclerosis

The axon (nerve fibre) is surrounded by a tube or sheath of myelin and the disease, multiple sclerosis, is characterised by patches or plaques of demyelination. The cause of the disease is unknown, as is the explanation for the patchy distribution of plaques. Initially there is an inflammatory or allergic reaction around the plaques. This usually subsides spontaneously and may be followed by remyelination. The scar formation in the nervous system is called gliosis and hardening of the plaques with time results in patches of sclerosis. The plaques seem to have a predilection for certain parts of the nervous system, in particular the optic nerves, the cerebellum, brain stem and spinal cord. They may also occur in the cerebral hemispheres, not infrequently in the later stages of the disease.

The disease usually starts in young adults between the ages of 20 and 45 but occasionally in the late teens, and less frequently in middle age. Females are affected more than males in the ratio of 3:2 and the incidence of the disease varies in different parts of the world, being commoner in temperate climates. In England the prevalence is about 40 per 100,000 but there is a tendency for clusters of cases to occur in certain areas.

Usually the disease is characterised by relapses and remissions, so a plaque may develop first in an optic nerve (*optic neuritis*) causing sudden loss of vision in one eye with recovery after a few weeks. The spontaneous recovery (remission) may then be followed by another relapse, e.g. a plaque in the spinal cord causing paraplegia. Plaques occur either singly in various parts of the nervous system at different times, or in crops. Recovery from each relapse may take several weeks or months but remissions can last for months, years or life. In about 25% of cases the course is relatively benign and the prognosis is good in that there is little or no permanent restriction of activities. In others after each successive relapse, there tends to be less recovery and thus more severe and persistent disability, and in about 20% of cases the disease is progressive.

The plaques involving the cerebellum or its brain stem connections cause a variety of cerebellar signs which may include nystagmus, titubation, clumsiness of the hands with intention tremor, and ataxia of gait. Speech becomes slurred, typically with a scanning or staccato type of dysarthria. Manifestations of the disease affecting other parts of the nervous system are frequently present at the same time or occur in subsequent relapses. These include visual and sensory symptoms, vertigo, loss of bladder control and upper motor neurone signs due to plaques in the spinal cord.

There is as yet no specific cure, but physiotherapy is usually advocated, and treatment with A.C.T.H. during acute relapses may enhance remission.

For further details of the disorders of the cerebellum see Table 8.

DISORDERS OF THE CEREBRAL CORTEX

Dysarthria occasionally results from lesions of the premotor area, which exerts cerebral control over the muscles of the face and those used for speech. This may be associated with motor or expressive dysphasia, and is called apraxic or cortical dysarthria. It results from the same pathological conditions which cause motor dysphasia (see Chapter 9) and from general paralysis of the insane (see page 130).

CHAPTER 12
DYSPHONIA

Dysphonia is weakness or hoarseness of the voice due to any lesion interfering with the laryngeal mechanism which governs voice production. There are a variety of non-neurological causes, the commonest of which is a sore throat with inflammation of the larynx (laryngitis). Hysteria is also a well-known cause of dysphonia. This is a functional disturbance without structural defect, often a reaction to an emotional upset, particularly in females. These patients usually just whisper and the lack of any true laryngeal disorder is usually evident as they can cough normally. Sudden spontaneous recovery takes place when psychological equilibrium is restored.

Patients with a tracheostomy are aphonic as the tube in the trachea prevents the expired air from reaching the larynx. Tumours and local lesions of the larynx also cause dysphonia and the voice tends to become deep and husky in patients with hypothyroidism (myxoedema).

The neuromuscular causes of Dysphonia

The mechanism of phonation is dependent on the muscles of the vocal cords supplied by the 10th cranial (vagus) nerves (see page 60). The adductors and tensors of the vocal colds contract on phonation and the abductors on inspiration. The vocal cords can be viewed by laryngoscopy and weakness of one or both results in dysphonia.

Dysphonia, like dysarthria, may be caused by the muscle diseases shown in Table 3. In some cases of myasthenia gravis (see page 56) there is excessive fatiguability of the laryngeal muscles which leads to increasing dysphonia, the voice becoming progressively weaker during the course of conversation. After a period of rest without talking or with drug therapy the voice may recover its strength only to fade again to a whisper after further talking and when the effects of treatment have worn off. This laryngeal fatiguability may be accentuated if accompanied by weakness of the respiratory muscles.

Dysphonia may also be due to lower motor neurone disorders. Those involving the vagus nerve or its branches are shown in Table 4a.

The recurrent laryngeal nerve or the vagus is particularly prone to damage in the neck and chest by:

(1) surgery—during thyroidectomy
(2) carcinoma of the thyroid
(3) carcinoma of the bronchus and malignant mediastinal growths
(4) aortic aneurysm

Occasionally unilateral vocal cord palsy is an isolated phenomenon and full investigations fails to reveal the cause. Some of these idiopathic cases may be due to a virus mononeuropathy of the vagus or recurrent laryngeal nerve.

A uniltaral recurrent laryngeal nerve lesion causes paralysis of the vocal cord; the resulting weakness of the voice may be slight and transient due to compensatory movement by the opposite vocal cord. With partial lesions of the recurrent laryngeal nerve, the abductors are always affected before the adductors (Semon's law) and therefore paralysis of adduction cannot occur without paralysis of abduction.

The sequence followed with a progressive lesion is abductor paralysis, midline position of the vocal cord due to overaction of the adductors, 'cadaveric' (intermediate) position and finally compensatory crossing over of the paralysed cord to a paramedian position.

Partial lesions causing bilateral abductor palsies produce laryngeal stridor (a harsh sound from the larynx) during inspiration. Total bilateral paralysis of the vocal cords causes complete aphonia so that the patient can only whisper.

The proximal part of the vagus nerve may be involved in the 'jugular foramen syndrome' in which the 9th, 10th and 11th cranial nerves are affected on one side. This may be caused by lesions at the base of the skull, such as a carcinoma spreading from the nasopharynx.

The lower motor neurone disorders involving the nuclei of the vagus in the medulla are shown in Table 4b, and dysphonia is part of the syndrome of bulbar palsy, as has been described in Chapter 10.

Dysphonia is also one of the features of pseudo-bulbar palsy, resulting from the disorders of upper motor neurones (bilaterally) as shown in Table 6.

Of the extra-pyramidal disorders shown in Table 7, dysphonia occurs most commonly in Parkinsonism, when the voice tends to be weak and monotonous. Dysphonia is rarely associated with cerebellar lesions, unless these involve the brain stem as well.

The clinical features and prognosis of neurological (paralytic) dysphonia are dependent on:

1. the mode of onset, i.e. acute or chronic
2. the position of the paralysed vocal cord
3. structural changes in the vocal cord, e.g. atrophy
4. anatomical variations in larynx, e.g. shape of glottis, position of arytenoids
5. compensation of non-paralysed cord
6. emotional reactions

Recovery, dependent, on the aetiology, can be divided into five stages:

1. *Aphonia*

Following an acute lesion of the recurrent laryngeal nerve, e.g. after thyroidectomy, the patient's voice may be completely lost (aphonia). Noises produced are rough, hoarse, and weak and the patient appears breathless because the period of phonation is reduced, producing rapid breathing (tachypnoea).

2. *Severe dysphonia*

Better glottal closure is obtained by compensatory moulding of the cartilages but this is less evident in the elderly (because of calcification).

3. *Flutter voice*

With further recovery, the different positions of the two vocal cords produce double tones (diplophony). In some cases, higher tones are lost resulting in a monotonous voice whereas in others, when the glottis is not completely closed, it becomes oval-shaped and results in a high-pitched falsetto.

4. *Mild dysphonia*

The volume of the voice increases and the hoarseness is compensated.

5. *Full recovery*

Full recovery is dependent on the aetiology and whether residual mobility of the vocal cord has been affected by structural changes.

PART 2

CHAPTER 13
CONGENITAL MALFORMATIONS
AND CEREBRAL PALSY

Congenital malformations are defined as abnormalities of structure present at birth. Infant mortality has decreased since the beginning of the century from 130 to nearly 20 per thousand live births; this progress is a reflection of improvements in ante-natal and obstetrical care together with advances in medical treament of neonatal disorders. The number of children with congential diseases has not changed so that they now provide a considerably higher proportion of neonatal mortality: whereas in 1900, 1/30 of the neonatal mortality was due to congenital abnormalities, now the proportion is approximately 1/4.

The incidence of congenital malformations depends on what is taken to be a malformation, whether still births are included and the age at which the incidence is assessed; approximately 1·5% at birth, it increases to 5% at one year of age. The C.N.S. is the commonest system affected by congenital malformation, 50% of all congenital lesions being neurological. Of 15 cases with congenital abnormalities, three will have spina-bifida, two anencephaly, two hydrocephalus, two heart disease, two cleft palate, and two mongolism, (the next commonest are club feet and dislocation of the hip): at least 7 of the 15 have C.N.S. involvement, or more if any of the cases of mongolism are mentally defective or retarded, as they often are. Other congenital conditions associated with mental defects include microcephaly and agenesis of the corpus callosum.

AETIOLOGY OF CONGENITAL
MALFORMATIONS

The causes may be environmental or genetic.

A Environmental causes acting on the foetus via the mother include:

   (1) dietary lack, either of protein, vitamin A, riboflavin, folic acid or thiamine
   (2) hormonal deficiency, e.g. of pituitary, thyroid or pancreas

(3) drugs, e.g. thalidomide, cortisone, antibiotics, nitrogen mustard, anticonvulsants

(4) physical agents, e.g. radiation, hypoxia, hyperthermia

(5) infections, e.g. rubella (german measles), toxoplasmosis, syphilis

B Genetic causes include chromosome mutation which may affect many systems (e.g. mongolism) and gene mutation which usually affects only one system.

The type of congenital defect depends on the stage of development of the foetus when the damage occurs. Severe malformation of the C.N.S. such as anencephaly, hydrocephalus and spina bifida cystica occur in about 1/150 births.

Anencephaly is due to a defect of the closure of the embryological neural tube, the brain is virtually absent, and this is usually incompatible with life. It occurs in females more than males in the proportion of 5:1 and is often associated with an absence of the ganglion cells of the retina. There is a geographical variation in incidence, e.g. it is three times commoner in Ireland than in London.

Hydrocephalus is due to excessive accumulation of cerebro-spinal fluid (C.S.F.) within the cranial cavity and occurs in about 1/1000 births.

The C.S.F. is formed by the choroid plexuses, which consist of a mass of tangled capillaries and lie in the lateral, third and fourth ventricles. By a process of selective perfusion and filtration, the C.S.F. is produced from the plasma in the choroid plexuses, passes through the foramina in the roof of the fourth ventricle into the subarachnoid space, and is absorbed via the arachnoid villi into the dural venous sinuses.

Hydrocephalus is described as *obstructive* if the circulation of the C.S.F. is blocked in the third ventricle, aqueduct or fourth ventricle; an example is aqueduct stenosis (which can be inherited in a sex-linked recessive manner). The lateral ventricles dilate and the cerebral cortex becomes thin.

Communicating hydrocephalus occurs when the C.S.F. is not adequately absorbed from the subarachnoid space, which may be due to adhesions following meningitis.

The head circumference is normally 33·1 cm at birth, 36·8 cm at one month, 39·4 cm at two months and 46·8 cm at a year. A hydrocephalic head is abnormally large and globular in shape with protuberance of the forehead, bulging fontanelles and prominent scalp veins. There is a cracked-pot note on percussion of the skull. These are the effects of excessive C.S.F. under high pressure, occurring before the sutures of the baby's skull have fused. About 50% of cases arrest spontaneously and 25% reach adult life. The average I..Q of hydrocephalics is 70, but 10% have an I.Q. above average. One-third have no physical disability, but the others tend to have squints or various degrees of spasticity. Frequently there are other associated abnormalities present as well, e.g. an Arnold-Chiari malformation (i.e. prolongation of the cerebellar vermis and tonsils with lengthened medulla), or spina bifida cystica, and in these complicated cases the prognosis is worse.

Microcephaly (abnormal smallness of the head and brain) also occurs in approximately 1/1000 births; it is always associated with mental deficiency, and a third of the cases have epilepsy. Similar complications are associated with agenesis of the corpus callosum. The development of language functions are likely to be delayed, or will remain retarded and immature when there are severe mental and intellectual defects.

CEREBRAL PALSY

Cerebral palsy is not a disease entity but is the term used to cover a variety of neurological disorders which result from maldevelopment of, or damage to, the brain and present at the time of birth or early infancy. The abnormalities of brain function are reflected most obviously by defects of movement, failure of development of intellect, speech and language in the widest sense, and disturbances of behaviour and emotional control. In many of the children affected, the limbs are stiff and there are pyramidal signs; this is the group often referred to as 'spastics'. In 10% of cases involuntary movements of an athetoid type—and not spasticity—constitute the principal disability, while in about 5% of cases, the limbs are actually hypotonic and the child may be ataxic rather than spastic.

The incidence is approximately 7 per 100,000 births; of these one dies in infancy, two are mentally defective, one is severely handicapped, two can be rehabilitated, and one has only mild disability. It is the latter two groups that are most important from the point of view of speech therapy. Between 1 and 2 of every 1000 school children have some form of cerebral palsy.

AETIOLOGY OF CEREBRAL PALSY

A. Pre-natal

1. Effect of maternal disorders on foetus in utero:
    (a) anaemia or toxaemia of pregnancy
    (b) infections transmitted from mother, e.g. rubella (german measles), toxoplasmosis, syphilis
    (c) rhesus incompatibility
2. Other embryological defects:
    (a) agenesis
    (b) porencephaly

B. Peri-natal

1. Prematurity
2. Birth trauma
3. Asphyxia, due to prolonged labour or difficult delivery

C. Post-natal

1. Infection, e.g. encephalitis
2. Cerebral venous thrombosis

The proportion of children with cerebral palsy due to birth trauma has probably declined and more attention has been focussed on the possibility of agenesis or hypogenesis, i.e. a failure of development of part of the brain which occurs for reasons usually unknown. Anoxia during or shortly after delivery accounts for some cases.

Rubella (german measles) if contracted by the mother during the first three months of pregnancy, is particularly liable to cause congenital malformations.

During embryonic life, the primitive organs go through phases of rapid development at different times, during which they are vulnerable to infection. The stage of development of the foetus at the time of infection will determine which embryological structures are likely to sustain maximum damage and, presumably, the severity of virulence of the infection is also significant. The common congenital malformations which result from rubella are deafness, congenital heart disease, abnormalities of the eyes, and occasionally more serious defects such as anencephaly.

Rhesus incompatibility may cause serious defects of the foetus. This is dependent upon the mother being rhesus negative and forming antibodies which on mixing with the foetal circulation, interfere with the maturation of foetal red blood cells resulting in varying degrees of *erythroblastosis foetalis*. The effects range from anaemia to severe degrees of jaundice which may produce *kernicterus* where bile pigment is deposited in the basal ganglia, and sometimes more diffusely throughout the brain, causing the ganglionic athetoid type of cerebral palsy, often with mental deficiency and deafness. The level of maternal antibodies increases with succeeding pregnancies so that the degree of erythroblastosis increases with each baby born; two or more such pregnancies may result in a miscarriage or still-birth.

CLINICAL TYPES OF CEREBRAL PALSY

Although cerebral palsy usually reveals itself by a delay in development with failure to pass the intellectual and physical milestones at the appropriate age, most cases fall into a number of distinctive clinical syndromes.

(a) Spastic

This is the commonest variety of cerebral palsy with upper motor neurone signs affecting the limbs, e.g. spastic diplegia (Little's disease), monoplegia, hemiplegia or double hemiplegia; this may be associated with mental defect varying from slight mental retardation to amentia and many of these cases develop epilepsy.

The mildest cases show a delay of a few months in learning to walk with some clumsiness and unsteadiness of gait, symmetrical exaggeration of the lower limb reflexes and extensor plantar responses. Often the child is unable to walk until the 5th or 6th year and then does so with a characteristic 'scissors gait' due to spasticity of the adductor muscles; contractures tend to develop in the tendo-Achilles and posterior thigh muscles. In the most severe case, walking never becomes possible and all four limbs are spastic, indicating bilateral or diffuse involvement of cortico-spinal pathways.

If the left cerebral hemisphere is maldeveloped or damaged, the right hemisphere may become dominant, leading to 'pathological' left-handedness. Language function may develop normally, e.g. if taken over by the right cerebral hemisphere, but in some cases speech development is retarded and there may be specific language disorders (see Chapter 6). With diffuse bilateral cortical damage causing amentia, speech and language functions may fail to develop.

Dysarthria is either due to a localised cortical defect causing articulatory apraxia or more commonly to pseudo-bulbar palsy resulting from bilateral involvement of cortico-bulbar fibres.

(b) Athetoid

This is sometimes called the ganglionic or extrapyramidal type due to involvement of the basal ganglia or other parts of the extrapyramidal system. It produces disorders of tone and posture with involuntary movements, e.g. athetosis or choreo-athetosis. These movements are not apparent until the 2nd year of life or even later, although the limbs are hypotonic and movement is inco-ordinate. Some cases have associated spasticity.

Speech in these cases is grossly distorted with an explosive dysarthria; there may also be dysphonia or interference with intonation and facial grimacing.

(c) Ataxic

This type is due to involvement of the cerebellar hemispheres and produces various degrees of inco-ordination and hypotonia, often with nystagmus. The speech disorder is due to an ataxic dysarthria.

Various combinations of the above clinical types occur, and there may be associated defects, e.g. deafness (which occurs in about 25% of cases, most commonly in the athetoid group), strabismus or other visual defects.

The age at which the diagnosis is made depends upon the severity of the condition, but it is usually within the first 12 to 18 months of life; in others, delay and difficulty in walking are not apparent until later in the 2nd year. The diagnosis of mental defect in early life, depending as it does on failure to achieve new milestones of intellectual development at the normal age (e.g. smiling, following a light, groping for objects, forming syllables and words etc.) requires experience because of normal variations.

Although a large proportion of patients with cerebral palsy are mentally defective, this is not invariable since gross neurological (e.g. motor) deficits can occur with little or no impairment of mental or intellectual processes. Furthermore, some children with cerebral palsy have specific defects of motor function (apraxia), of sensory function (agnosia), of the special senses (e.g. nerve deafness) or of speech and language ('aphasia', articulatory apraxia, dyslexia—see Chapter 6); these can give a false impression of mental defect if clinical appraisal is superficial or limited. Thus specific defects of speech and other language functions are sometimes misdiagnosed as mental deficiency. However if there is a discrepancy between basic intelligence and language function due to defects predominantly in the sphere of speech and language, then attempts should be made to compensate for the specific disorder by special methods of individual training either of the defective function or of the unaffected functions. It is very important that these children, as well as those with specific non-language disorders (as above), are recognised and educated appropriately; although requiring patient individual training, many can be helped considerably.

In some cases, motor disorders can be alleviated by surgical methods so helping these children to lead useful lives, but the prognosis will be poor if there are severe intellectual and motor deficits.

INFANTILE HEMIPLEGIA

Infantile hemiplegia can be present from birth (congenital hemiplegia) when it may be due to a cystic deformity of one cerebral hemisphere (porencephaly) or to infarction of the brain occurring in utero. More commonly it develops acutely in infancy or early childhood, often during the course of an acute infection such as whooping cough or following a 'febrile convulsion'. Probably the most common cause is cerebral infarction from arterial or venous occlusion, resulting in scarring and atrophy of the cerebral hemisphere with localised dilatation of the lateral ventricle.

The affected arm is severely paralysed, finger and hand movements being abolished and the hand and forearm assume a typically flexed posture lying across the front of the chest. The leg, though spastic with exaggerated deep reflexes and an extensor plantar response, is less severely affected and all patients are eventually able to walk, often with surprisingly little difficulty.

Infantile hemiplegia is rarely bilateral; it can then be distinguished from a spastic diplegia due to cerebral palsy (Little's disease) by the fact that in infantile hemiplegia the upper limbs are more severely affected than the lower.

If the dominant hemisphere is involved after speech has developed, aphasia results; the earlier the age of the child the more complete and rapid is the recovery of speech function. If the dominant hemisphere is involved before speech is acquired, the development of speech may be delayed; and in some cases speech function becomes established in the opposite hemisphere.

Residual neurological deficits can be of all grades of severity, but are sometimes only trivial. In the more severe cases, epilepsy is a common complication as the scar in the affected hemisphere acts as an irritative focus. In those cases in which epileptic seizures are frequent and severe, brain damage is marked and intellectual impairment and behaviour disorders are common.

CHAPTER 14

EPILEPSY

Epilepsy is one of the important manifestations of brain disease and epileptic attacks occasionally cause transient disturbances of speech without loss of consciousness. The study of epilepsy is particularly helpful in understanding brain function.

The term epilepsy is used to describe recurrent disturbances of consciousness, movement, feeling or behaviour which are primarily cerebral in origin. Such attacks take the form of fits or seizures, often but not always with convulsions. Epilepsy is called *idiopathic* when the cause is not known, and *symptomatic* if due to local or diffuse disease of the brain. Attacks resembling epilepsy, sometimes with convulsions, can also result from fainting due to a fall in blood pressure (syncope), or a fall in blood sugar (hypoglycaemia) or in blood calcium (hypocalcaemia), but the diagnosis in these cases depends on the nature of the underlying systemic disorder.

Epileptic attacks are paroxysmal, repetitive, usually stereotyped and cease spontaneously. The susceptibility or threshold to fits varies in different individuals, and may vary in the same individual at different times. Genetic or constitutional factors influence the liability to develop epilepsy, some brains being more susceptible. There is a wide range of factors which provoke fits.

The threshold for fits is lowered by hyperventilation and photic stimulation and both these are used routinely during recording of the electroencephalogram (E.E.G.); other metabolic disturbances may have

TABLE 9. Factors provoking fits

Hyperventilation
Photic and other reflex stimuli
Stress, anxiety, depression, sleep
Other metabolic factors
   e.g. overhydration, premenstrual state,
   hypoglycaemia, hypoxia, fever,
   withdrawl of drugs, etc.
Structural brain lesions—diffuse and focal

---

the same effect. Even in a healthy person a potent stimulus, e.g. an electric shock or analeptic drug will produce a convulsion. The list of provoking factors includes structural brain lesions, such as a cerebral tumour, abscess, or penetrating brain wound, but less than 50% of patients with these lesions develop epilepsy. This suggests that there are inhibiting factors preventing clinical attacks, as does the fact that a small proportion of people have E.E.G.s with epileptic activity, yet do not have fits.

About 4 or 5 per thousand of the adult population have epilepsy so that in England and Wales there are approximately a quarter of a million people with epilepsy. Considering the enormous amount of electrical activity in the brain, it is perhaps surprising that epilepsy is not more common.

AETIOLOGY

(a) *Idiopathic:* When the pathological cause of attacks is not known, the term idiopathic epilepsy is used. This may be due to disturbances of cell metabolism that cannot be defined by present techniques of investigation. However the E.E.G. in idiopathic epilepsy typically shows paroxysms of abnormal generalised excessive electrical discharges, probably originating centrally, either from structures deep in the cerebral hemispheres or from the reticular substance of the brain stem. This type of idiopathic epilepsy is also called centrencephalic epilepsy. Some factors predisposing to the development of idiopathic epilepsy are genetically determined (i.e. inherited) and account for the familial incidence of epilepsy. Idiopathic epileptic attacks usually begin between the ages of 2 and 20, although the onset is sometimes later.

Epilepsy can also result from defects of development or damage of the brain before birth, i.e. while the foetus is still in utero, or from injury to the brain during parturition.

(b) *Symptomatic:* Epilepsy, if not idiopathic, is a symptom of a cerebral lesion occurring in a patient with an inborn susceptibility. There are many causes of symptomatic epilepsy, some of which are shown in Table 10. Focal attacks in adults are nearly always indicative of symptomatic epilepsy. Any form of epilepsy developing after the age of 20 is referred to as 'epilepsy of late onset' to indicate that it may be symptomatic and requires special investigation. Only about 20% of these cases do in fact have a cerebral tumour, and some of the remainder will turn out to have idiopathic epilepsy in spite of the relatively late age of onset. Epilepsy—like headache—should be regarded as a symptom; it is not a single disease entity.

TABLE 10. Aetiology of epilepsy

Idiopathic	Centrencephalic
	Cryptogenic
Symptomatic	Tumours
	Infective, e.g. encephalitis
	abscess
	neurosyphilis
	Cerebral infarction
	Angioma
	Trauma
	Toxic and degenerative diseases

CLASSIFICATION OF EPILEPTIC ATTACKS

There are many different types of epilepsy and, quite apart from the variety of causes, as mentioned in the preceding paragraphs, epileptic attacks may be classified according to the clinical features, and the E.E.G. findings; these should be correlated when possible.

The two main types of epileptic attacks are (1) generalised and (2) focal.

TABLE 11. Classification of epileptic attacks

1. Generalised	(a) grand mal
	(b) petit mal
	(c) status epilepticus
2. Focal	(a) Jacksonian
	(b) temporal lobe
	(c) epilepsia partialis continuans

1. GENERALISED EPILEPTIC ATTACKS

These are divided into (a) grand mal and (b) petit mal, names given by French neurologists who first described them.

(a) Grand mal

A grand mal attack produces sudden loss of consciousness with or without a warning. The warning or aura is transient, lasts only a few seconds and ranges from a vague feeling of faintness or giddiness to a variety of phenomena depending on the part of the cerebral cortex in which the discharge begins. The aura is followed by loss of consciousness, and the patient may fall and injure himself. There is often a sudden cry due to the involuntary expulsion of air through the closed glottis indicating the start of the *tonic phase*, i.e. sustained contraction of the body with the arms and legs held rigidly in flexion or extension. During this stage the tongue may be bitten, the patient makes gurgling, groaning or choking sounds, froths at the mouth and becomes cyanosed from asphyxia. The tonic phase lasts for about half a minute and is followed by the *clonic phase*, i.e. alternating contractions of the extensor and flexor muscles of the limbs causing rhythmical repetitive jerking movements, i.e. convulsions. This phase usually lasts for a few minutes during which incontinence of urine (involuntary micturition) may take place. This is followed by the *post-ictal state* when the patient may complain of headache, muscular pains and nausea and there may be a period of confusion or sleep lasting from a few minutes to hours; sometimes actions are performed without being remembered (automatism). Not all grand mal seizures follow the same pattern, for example, the clonic phase may be very short, or absent i.e. without convulsive movements, or there may merely be a short bout of muscular twitching.

The E.E.G. in idiopathic grand mal typically shows paroxysms of high voltage discharges bilaterally and synchronously from both cerebral hemispheres. Grand mal attacks may thus have an idiopathic (centrencephalic) basis, but can also be symptomatic of structural cerebral lesions.

(b) Petit mal

Petit mal attacks are characterised by a momentary absence in which the mind goes blank and the child's expression appears vacant. This lasts for a matter of a few seconds or less and the eyes usually remain open and stare. The child may feel giddy, become pale or flushed, lose the thread of conversation, drop things or even fall momentarily but recovery is rapid. These attacks can occur several times a day and when very frequent, for example 100 per day, the name *pyknolepsy* is given.

The E.E.G. in petit mal has a characteristic pattern with high voltage bilaterally synchronous discharges of spike-and-wave complexes recurring regularly at 3 cycles per second (Fig. 6d). This E.E.G. picture differentiates true petit mal from other forms of minor epilepsy where loss of consciousness is also incomplete or momentary but due to focal cerebral disturbances. Petit mal almost invariably begins in childhood and is idiopathic.

2. FOCAL EPILEPTIC ATTACKS

Focal attacks are due to a local lesion of the brain. The disturbances of brain function depend upon the situation of the lesion, and the attacks consist of transient excitatory or inhibitory phenomena. If the lesion is progressive, this will lead to permanent neurological deficits.

Focal electrical discharges can remain localised but sometimes spread over the cortex and trigger off abnormal electrical activity in contiguous areas. This spread or 'march' of epileptic activity is reflected clinically; for example, attacks may begin with tingling on the right side of the face, spread to the right hand up the right arm and down the right side of the body to the leg, possibly followed by motor phenomena with twitching or jerking movements of the muscles of the right side of the body. This indicates a spread of the electrical discharge from the face area of the sensory cortex spreading upwards over the post-central gyrus and going on to involve the motor cortex. This type of focal attack with its sequential spread or march is called *Jacksonian epilepsy* (after Hughlings Jackson). The focal discharge can spread extensively, become generalised and precipitate a grand mal attack. The aura is important because it localises the epileptogenic focus, e.g. an aura of jerking of the right leg would indicate a lesion irritating the parasagittal premotor region of the left hemisphere; an aura of a peculiar smell or taste indicates a temporal lobe lesion (see later). If there is no aura because the electrical discharge very rapidly becomes generalised with loss of consciousness, or if the patient fails to remember the aura subsequently, evidence of a focal origin may still be obtained from investigations, for example, an electrical focus may be found on the E.E.G., or a cerebral tumour or angioma demonstrated by X-rays.

Temporal Lobe Epilepsy

This is a form of focal epilepsy where attacks originate from an abnormality in the temporal lobe; if the focus lies in the temporal lobe of the dominant hemisphere there may be an aura of dysphasia. There are often disturbances of memory, e.g. the patient may just for a few seconds relive experiences that occurred some time previously, or feel that he is seeing or doing something which seems familiar but which he may not have seen or done before (déjà-vu, déjà-fait phenomena); or everything may seem strange and unfamiliar when it is in fact well known to him (jamais-vu). Odd sensations known as 'dreamy states' may occur, as well as the feeling of not existing (depersonalisation and derealisation). *Uncinate attacks* consist of hallucinations of smell (olfactory) and taste (gustatory) usually lasting just a few seconds. These are due to a lesion of the uncus (the medial part of the temporal lobe); the patient is aware of a smell, often with a burning or musty nature or indescribable. With this or separately, he may experience a peculiar, indescribable or perhaps familiar taste.

Various other hallucinations also occur:

Auditory: the impression of hearing a sound, such as bells ringing, phrases from a musical theme or a voice which may or may not be familiar.

Vertiginous: the sensation of rotatory movement, either the head spinning or the room going round and round, similar to that experienced when getting off a roundabout.

Visual: formed hallucinations of vision may consist of remembered scenes, familiar objects, places, people or faces and all sorts of fictional images; there may be distortions of visual perception with micropsia, macropsia or apparent displacement of visual objects.

If visual hallucinations consist of crude (unformed) but stereotyped phenomena, for example, various shapes or abstract patterns which are not recognisable or remembered as particular objects, or flashing lights appearing in homonymous parts of the visual fields, then the epileptogenic focus is likely to be situated more posteriorly in the temporo-occipital region, closer to the calcarine (visual) cortex.

Attacks of temporal lobe epilepsy may thus consist of recurrent disturbances of speech or memory, or one of the above hallucinations, lasting for a few seconds at a time. Alternatively a transient disturbance of this type may be the aura of a grand mal epileptic attack and would indicate that the focus, i.e. the site of origin of the attack, was in one temporal lobe. However some auras resulting from focal lesions in the temporal lobe are less distinct consisting of abdominal sensations, sickly or sinking feelings in the stomach (visceral or epigastric aura) which pass up the body to the head and may be followed by loss of consciousness. In others there is just an indescribable sensation in the head (cephalic aura) or disturbances of behaviour (*psychomotor attacks*). Champing or sucking movements of the mouth are also manifestations of temporal lobe attacks.

STATUS EPILEPTICUS

A series of fits occasionally follow one another rapidly so that the patient has hardly recovered from one when the process is repeated (serial epilepsy). 'Status epilepticus' occurs when the fits recur repeatedly without any intervening recovery of consciousness. This is a very dangerous condition which may prove fatal so that all such cases should be admitted to hospital for appropriate treatment as soon as possible.

Focal fits which continue unabated for long periods are referred to as *epilepsia partialis continuans*.

SPEECH DISTURBANCES IN EPILEPSY

With petit mal, the attacks may interrupt the child's normal flow of speech, he may miss something that is said to him and lose the thread of conversation during the transient period of loss of awareness.

In temporal lobe epilepsy when the focus lies in the dominant hemisphere attacks may have a dysphasic aura; with an epileptogenic lesion in any part of the speech area, the attack itself may consist only of transient dysphasia or there may be a dysphasic aura preceding a grand mal seizure. The dysphasia may consist of any of the disturbances of speech and language described in Chapter 9, and such transient dysphasia—either alone or as the aura of a grand mal attack—is of great localising value indicating that a lesion lies in the speech area of the dominant cerebral hemisphere.

Dysphasia or hemiplegia discovered for the first time *after* an epileptic attack may be the result of the epileptogenic lesion, but such signs occurring post-ictally do not always have the same localising significance as the aura, as they may be due to an inhibitory effect of the fit (Todd's paralysis). Recovery from this usually takes place within a few days.

ELECTROENCEPHALOGRAPHY

Electrical activity in the human body is a reflection of the biochemical and metabolic processes of the individual cells. The electrical impulses from the brain were originally discovered by Berger, a German psychiatrist who published his first paper in 1929. These impulses can be recorded as the sum total of electrical activity of the 10,000 million cells of the cerebral cortex. The normal record consists of alpha or Berger rhythm of 9–11 cycles per second (Fig. 6a) which is recorded chiefly over the occipital areas. The alpha rhythm is more marked when the eyes are closed and becomes less prominent with the eyes open; this is referred to as blocking of the alpha rhythm.

Abnormalities in the E.E.G. may be generalised or focal and can be of diagnostic value. The diagnosis of epilepsy depends principally on the clinical features of the attacks but the E.E.G. may be of considerable help in differentiating different types of epilepsy.

In idiopathic (centrencephalic) epilepsy, the E.E.G. shows characteristic paroxysms of bilaterally synchronous sharp complexes of high voltage. Fig. 6c shows grand mal components and Fig. 6d spike-and-wave complexes of petit mal. These abnormalities may be provoked or exaggerated in some cases by hyperventilation, photic stimulation (flicker) and occasionally by various other special techniques.

The usual recording between seizures may lead to various diagnostic difficulties because over 10% of epileptics have a normal E.E.G. and about 10% of normal people (who have never had a fit) have an abnormal E.E.G. A normal E.E.G. does not exclude idiopathic epilepsy, nor symptomatic epilepsy, since even a patient with a cerebral tumour can have a normal E.E.G. Local lesions of the brain such as tumours or abscesses may be reflected by focal abnormalities in the E.E.G. (Fig. 6b) but as a rule no conclusion regarding the pathological nature of brain lesions can be made from the E.E.G. alone.

TREATMENT OF EPILEPSY

The main drugs now used in the treatment of epilepsy are listed in Table 12.

These are the drugs usually tried first, either singly or in various combinations. They are effective in preventing attacks in a large proportion of cases. Sometimes, however, alternative or additional

FIGURE 6. Electroencephalograms. (a) Normal record; alpha rhythm blocking when eyes opened. (b) Left posterior parietal tumour; focal abnormality with slow waves. (c) Centrencephalic epilepsy; bilateral spike discharges provoked by flicker. (d) Petit mal; 3 c/s spike and wave complexes.

TABLE 12. Drug treatment of epilepsy

Petit mal	Ethosuximide (Zarontin)
	Sodium Valproate (Epilim)
Grand mal and Focal	Phenobarbitone
	Phenytoin (Epanutin)
	Primidone (Mysoline)

treatment is required and a variety of other anticonvulsant drugs are available, e.g. carbamazepine (tegretol), sulthiame (ospolot), pheneturide (benuride), nitrazepam (mogadon) and clonazepam (rivotril).

Treatment of a grand mal attack

The patient should be prevented from doing any damage to himself or anybody else and should be allowed to lie in a space cleared of obstructions; any padding available such as cushions or blankets should be placed to prevent injury to the head and limbs during convulsions; no attempt need be made to restrain forcibly the convulsive movements. It may be possible to prevent the tongue from being bitten if something firm and padded is available to put between the teeth before they are clenched tightly. Force or fingers should not be used and it is worth remembering that the tongue will heal but broken teeth will not.

During the phase of unconsciousness, the airway has to be kept clear, dentures should be removed, the collar loosened and the patient turned on to his side or semi-prone. Recovery usually follows without any complication; if the dagnosis of epilepsy has been established previously it is seldom necessary to call a doctor or send the patient to hospital unless an injury has been sustained in the attack and requires treatment. Medical advice should be sought for the first fit, and a series of fits in quick succession or status epilepticus demands urgent hospital treatment.

Surgical treament of Epilepsy

If the causative lesion is, for example, a benign tumour, surgical removal may be possible and would offer a high chance of cure although epileptic attacks may still recur due to residual brain damage.

If the E.E.G. repeatedly shows a focal origin in an area of the brain which can be excised, for example, the anterior part of one frontal or temporal lobe, neurosurgical treatment is occasionally possible even when special X-ray investigations have failed to reveal a lesion.

Removal of the anterior 5–6 cm of the temporal lobe, sparing the superior temporal gyrus, is called *temporal lobectomy*. Such operations are suitable for a small proportion of those with temporal lobe epilepsy whose attacks prove resistant to medical treatment. Pathological examination of the removed tissue sometimes shows sclerosis or atrophy (shrinkage) with gliosis which is considered to be due to hypoxia resulting from birth trauma or prolonged convulsions in infancy.

CHAPTER 15
DEMENTIA

Dementia means deterioration of intellectual functions, so that there is impairment of memory, intelligence and a wide variety of aptitudes and accomplishments. The term has usually been used to imply an irreversible state as the conditions causing dementia were nearly always progressive or untreatable. This is no longer invariably the case, since several causes of dementia can now be treated effectively, e.g. benign intracranial tumours, neurosyphilis and Vitamin B12 deficiency. Early diagnosis of these treatable conditions is important as the degree of recovery depends largely on how early treatment is started. All patients with dementia therefore require investigation to establish the cause as soon as possible.

Dementia must be distinguished from amentia, which is the failure or impairment of intellectual development. Mental and intellectual faculties are dependent on the integrated and selective functions of the millions of cells in the cerebral cortex. The greatest degree of *learning* ability is in youth although, with experience and training, memory patterns and skills are established and judgement improves. During middle life, the cells of the cerebral cortex beign to dwindle, probably by more than a 100,000 each day. This is part of the natural process of ageing (physiological senescence) so that most old people do not have the same intellectual capacity as when they were young, the earliest sign being loss of memory for recent events with a tendency to become forgetful of names. Physiological senescence and senile dementia are not synonymous as dementia implies a pathological process.

If intellectual deterioration occurs before the age of 65, the term *presenile dementia* is used, but this serves only to indicate the relatively early age of onset as the pathological causes may be the same as in the elderly.

In any patient with dementia—whatever the cause—speech may be affected, but vocabulary may be retained until quite late in the illness. Although speech therapy will not help if there is a significant degree of dementia, it is important to be aware of the different types of altered speech observed and the pathological processes of the brain which interfere with the mental faculties.

Causes of Dementia

Dementia is not a diagnosis but a manifestation (cf. dysphasia and hemiplegia) of various diseases. The underlying cause has to be established, particularly so that the potentially reversible disorders are not overlooked; the classification shown in Table 13 is suggested.

TABLE 13. Causes of dementia

Metabolic Disorders
  Deficiency of Vitamin B_1 (Korsakoffs' psychosis, Wernicke's
                                  encephalopathy, see Chapter 3)
        Vitamin B_2 (Pellagra)
        Vitamin B_{12}
  Hypothyroidism
  Hypoglycaemia
  Hepatic and renal failure
  Drugs, e.g. barbiturates, alcohol, bromides
              arsenic, lead, mercury
  Cerebral anoxia, e.g. following cardiac arrest
  Lipidoses

Degenerative Diseases
  Alzheimer's, Pick's
  Huntington's chorea
  Jakob-Creutzfeldt disease (? due to slow virus)

Infections (see Chapter 18)
  Neurosyphilis

Hydrocephalus (see Chapter 13)
  Obstructive, Communicating

Tumours (see Chapter 16)
  e.g. of frontal lobes and corpus callosum

Trauma (see Chapter 19)
  Brain injuries
  'Punch drunk' syndrome
  Chronic subdural haematoma

The disruption of mental functions is often generalised (global dementia) and includes deterioration of intelligence, memory, behaviour and personality. Deficits can also be selective, so that formal intelligence may be preserved yet serious lapses of judgement occur.

The development of slovenliness may occasionally be an important early feature of dementia, but there is usually failure of memory and of the power of reasoning, lack of retention or recall, and loss of learning ability. Patients with chronic dementia may show both perseveration and confabulation. Confabulation is also seen in more severe cases of G.P.I. (see page 130). But the earliest presentation is often an inability to perform professional duties. Both Pick's disease and Alzheimer's disease are characterised by memory loss, with a reduction in vocabulary in the former and with disorientation in time and space in the latter.

Differentiation from psychosis, particularly depression, and occasionally schizophrenia may be difficult; focal cerebral lesions which cause frontal lobe disinhibition, dysphasia and parietal lobe syndromes with apraxia must also be distinguished.

Patients who complain that they have to write notes as they are unable to remember things, usually do not have any serious disease. Their subjective forgetfulness may not be confirmed by tests and may be due to an anxiety state or neurosis, often being associated with headache and lack of concentration. The patient with organic dementia in contrast, conceals or is unaware of his disability and, lacking insight and judgement, may have to be persuaded by friends or relatives to consult a doctor.

Patients with dementia may be dysphasic or depressed as well. If the dementia is severe, disorientation in time and place occurs, sometimes accompanied by delusions and hallucinations. In advanced cases, there may be epileptic attacks and a variety of neurological signs, often with incontinence. In some, there is apathy and withdrawal whereas in others, there is a general motor restlessness, confusion, emotional lability, psychotic and anti-social behaviour. The presenting features often seem to be dependent more on the pre-morbid personality than the pathological process.

Examination of the mental state

It is necessary to observe general behaviour, for example, relationship to other people and the response to situations and the surroundings.

Tests for memory and intellectual deterioration should include the assessment of orientation in space and time, simple arithmetical tests, such as 100 minus 7, sentence repetition, and tests of general knowledge.

Obviously these tests need to be geared to the intellectual background of the individual patient.

The patient's method of speaking as well as the content should be observed and sometimes taped, particularly spontaneous talk, which may be hesitant, slow, or discursive with sudden changes of topic.

The patient's mood and the presence of delusions or hallucinations should be noted, as well as whether the patient is orientated as to his own name, identity, place, time and date.

Memory for both recent and more remote experiences can also be assessed as can the grasp of general information, insight and judgement. The patient should be asked to write something in his own time, for example a brief account of a day in his life.

The Babcock sentence, 'There is one thing a nation must have to be rich and great, and that is a large, secure supply of wood', is a useful test. It is repeated alternately by the examiner and patient until the patient says it perfectly. Normally this is achieved within two or three attempts; failure after several attempts is indicative of dementia. Gross perseveration of an error is typical of an organic intellectual loss, and fragmentary repetition is suggestive of a language defect. Gross variability in response is often characteristic of psychoneurosis (Zangwill, 1943). The explanation of simple proverbs is another useful test.

Types of demented speech

Speech can be described in several ways, e.g. phonetic, phonemic, linguistic, syntactic or semantic. Patients with dementia show poverty of speech so that in severe cases the patient is inaccessible. Although all forms of language (speaking, writing and reading) are affected, expressive vocabulary of speech is most affected, a larger vocabulary being retained in writing and most with reading. There is difficulty in retaining series but, unlike aphasic patients, paraphasia, neologisms and portmanteaux words do not occur. Names for objects are often not completely accurate although they may have a close association. Interjections are rarely used although speech can be exclamatory. Speech is simplified consisting of statements, descriptions or requests, often of no importance.

It has been found that the ratio between the numbers of verbs and adjectives used varies, as in neurotics, and there is also variation in the length of sentences and punctuation. The frequency of the pronoun 'I' is also of interest: used in 5% of words over a telephone by a normal person it is used in 0·01% in technical speech. Both in dementia and aphasia sentences are started but not finished (aposiopesis) and there is filling in with unnecessary additions (paralogisms). Perseveration is extremely common; words are used normally but then reiterated (contamination) and this is also seen in writing (echographia). Echolalia is found in dementia as well as aphasia. In presenile dementias such as Pick's and Alzheimer's disease, speech is slow and there may be interpolation of the 's' and 't' sounds, and the voice also tends to become higher-pitched.

A demented patient has difficulty in understanding quick or noisy speech. Gesture, gesticulation, mime and mimicry may all be impaired, possibly in part due to slowness of movements (akinesia). The term *alogia* has been used for the impoverishment of speech in dementia; this differs from the purely communicative defects of dysphasia, which is due to a local cortical lesion of the specific area of the brain concerned with speech.

CHAPTER 16
TUMOURS

Pathology

Tumours are abnormal growths (neoplasms) and are classified as primary or secondary. A primary tumour consists of microscopic cells that are similar to those of the tissues in which it develops. These cells proliferate and the resulting tumour may be benign or malignant.

A *benign* tumour grows slowly, and does not infiltrate or invade locally or spread to other parts of the body. It thus remains confined to the structure of origin, is often encapsulated and its main effects are due to compression of surrounding tissues.

A *malignant* tumour infiltrates the tissues in which it develops and invades neighbouring structures; many malignant tumours metastasise, i.e. spread to other parts of the body, the malignant cells of the primary growth infiltrating into the lymphatic or blood circulation and so are transported to organs elsewhere. These cells then form secondary tumours or deposits (metastases) which continue to grow and spread in the same way. Secondary tumours are thus the result of the metastasis of primary malignant tumours and consist of cells similar to those of the primary tumour.

Tumour cells as seen under a microscope have characteristic shapes and patterns resembling the cells of the tissues from which they arise. The most malignant tumours consist of mainly primitive and poorly differentiated cells which tend to proliferate rapidly. Cell multiplication is the result of mitosis and the demonstration of mitotic cells under the microscope usually indicates that the tumour is malignant.

The names given to tumours (whether benign or malignant) frequently end in the suffix '-oma', e.g. meningioma, astrocytoma—the first part of the name indicating the structure or type of cells from which the tumour originates. The suffix '-blastoma' implies that the tumour is composed of blast or primitive cells which are usually highly malignant. Some malignant tumours are referred to as carcinoma (e.g. of bronchus or breast) and these are amongst the most common forms of cancer.

INTRACRANIAL TUMOURS

Primary intracranial tumours originate from the structures within the skull, e.g. the meninges (*meningioma*) or within the brain (e.g. *glioma*). The secondary intracranial tumours (metastases) originate from a primary growth elsewhere in the body, usually a carcinoma of the lung or breast.

The clinical manifestations of intracranial tumours include:

(1) the general effects of raised intracranial pressure, i.e. headache, vomiting and papilloedema,

(2) local symptoms and signs, dependent on the site of the tumour and on its rate of growth, and

(3) epilepsy, focal or generalised, if one or both cerebral hemispheres are involved.

These may occur singly or in any combination.

Meningioma

This is a primary tumour of the meninges and can develop in the spinal canal as well as intracranially; it is more common in women.

Meningiomas are benign tumours, i.e. they grow relatively slowly, do not actively infiltrate the brain and do not metastasise. The local effects are due to direct compression or displacement of the brain in which they may become deeply embedded. Raised intracranial pressure eventually develops and, if not relieved, death will ensue. These tumours usually grow into spherical shaped or irregular, lobulated masses with a relatively small point of attachment where the tumour originated from the dura, but sometimes they extend as a solid layer (meningioma en plaque). They may also produce thickening of the overlying bone (hyperostosis) and occasionally erode through the skull to form a palpable or visible swelling on the head. There is a predilection for certain sites so that the symptoms and signs will vary with the structures involved.

(1) *Olfactory groove* meningioma will compress or displace the olfactory nerve and cause loss of the sense of smell (anosmia). As it increases in size it may compress the optic nerve causing loss of vision with primary optic atrophy. Raised intracranial pressure may supervene with generalised headache, vomiting and papilloedema. Olfactory groove meningiomas also compress the frontal lobes of the cerebral

hemispheres causing changes in personality, behaviour and mood, often with disinhibition and mental and intellectual deterioration. Tumours in this situation can present with various types of epilepsy including status epilepticus.

If the frontal lobe of the dominant cerebral hemisphere is involved and the tumour impinges on the speech area, this will cause dysphasia. A monoparesis or hemiplegia eventually develops with a grasp reflex, i.e. the hand grasps involuntarily or reflexly anything that touches the palm. This is a primitive reflex seen normally during the first few months of life in infants, who grasp a finger or other object placed across the palm and do not let go unless forced to do so. Another manifestation of frontal lobe lesions is loss of control of micturition, usually with incontinence.

(2) *Parasagittal* or *convexity* meningioma originates from the falx near the sagittal sinus or the dura mater over the convexity of the cerebral hemispheres. Parasagittal meningioma may present with focal epilepsy starting in the opposite foot with transient motor or sensory disturbances which later become persistent and progressive.

(3) *Sphenoidal ridge* meningioma arises from the region of the greater or lesser wing of the sphenoid bone. The tumour enlarges in the middle fossa to compress the temporal lobe causing temporal lobe epilepsy (see Chapter 14). If the tumour is on the side of the dominant cerebral hemisphere, dysphasia develops. Involvement of the lower fibres of the optic radiation will produce contralateral homonymous upper quadrantic visual field defects, progressing to a complete homonymous hemianopia if the whole of the optic radiation becomes involved.

(4) *Parasellar* meningioma occurs around the pituitary fossa. The tumour presses on the optic nerves, chiasm or tracts, causing the corresponding visual field defects and primary optic atrophy.

(5) *Tentorial* meningioma arises from the tentorium cerebelli and grows either in a supra-tentorial direction compressing one or both cerebral hemispheres, or downwards (infra-tentorially) into the posterior fossa compressing the cerebellum or brain stem. In the latter case there will be signs of cerebellar dysfunction, which may include dysarthria (see Chapter 11).

The diagnosis of a meningioma may sometimes be suspected if the plain X-rays of the skull show a localised area of erosion or sclerosis of the bone overlying the tumour. Arteriography may show displacement of vessels by the tumour, which typically shows a 'radiological blush' due to its vascularity (the blush resulting from filling of the tumour blood vessels with the radiopaque dye).

Many meningiomas can be completely removed and the prognosis is usually good. Operation relieves the raised intracranial pressure, the focal neurological signs regress and may clear completely if the damage has not been too severe or long standing. Epileptic attacks also cease unless there has been irreversible damage of the cerebral cortex by the tumour prior to removal. Because the tumour may have interfered with the blood supply to part of the brain, neurological disability may prove to be permanent. It is not always possible to remove the tumour completely so that, some time after operation, the signs recur due to regrowth of the remaining tumour. This occasionally takes on a more rapidly growing form with less differentiated cells (meningiosarcoma). Because of the danger of recurrence, radiotherapy may be advised postoperatively.

Dysphasia results from a meningioma pressing on the speech area, and dysarthria from a posterior fossa meningioma involving the brain stem or cerebellum; these speech disorders, like the other effects, will be progressive unless the tumour is removed. Post-operative speech therapy may help to enhance recovery of language function and compensate for residual defects. Various factors influence the prognosis for recovery of speech (see Chapter 9).

Glioma

Gliomas are more common than meningiomas. Gliomas are primary malignant tumours of the brain originating from the glial cells, i.e. astrocytes, oligodendrocytes and microglia which form the connective tissue of the brain. These tumours are named according to the microscopic appearances of the cells.

The commonest type of glioma is an *astrocytoma* which is derived from cells of the astrocyte type. These tumours are locally malignant and infiltrate the brain substance but do not metastasise outside the nervous system. The rate of growth and spread of astrocytomas vary and different grades of malignancy can be recognised microscopically. These grades are numbered 1–4, the most malignant being grade 4 and called glioblastoma multiforme or spongioblastoma. These latter types are recognised by the presence of undifferentiated primitive cells frequently seen in mitosis. Tumours of this type often present with epilepsy, symptoms and signs of raised intracranial pressure, and focal neurological deficits. There is progressive deterioration leading to death often within a few months from the onset of symptoms. On the other hand grade 1 astrocytoma can be very slow growing, the first indication of a cerebral lesion (e.g. a focal fit) occurring sometimes as long as 5, 10 or even 15 years before death.

Oligodendrogliomas are derived from the oligodendrocytes, and usually grow very slowly. Like the slow-growing astrocytomas, calcification often occurs in them and can be seen radiologically.

The prognosis with gliomas is usually poor since infiltration of the brain substance prevents removal of all of the tumour, which probably extends further than is obvious to the naked eye at operation. Complete removal and cure is occasionally achieved, e.g. if an astrocytoma grade 1 is diagnosed early and removed in toto by temporal lobectomy. Sometimes, large cysts form within an astrocytoma, fill up with fluid and cause raised intracranial pressure. These can be aspirated with relief of pressure symptoms. The more malignant gliomas form many abnormal blood vessels so that the tumour is very vascular. Haemorrhages are then liable to occur spontaneously or on attempted biopsy (i.e. surgical removal of a small piece of tumour for diagnostic microscopic examination). Although radiotherapy is given in some cases, the results are not very encouraging as these tumours are rarely radiosensitive.

Other cerebral tumours

Ependymoma are tumours derived from the ependymal cells which line the ventricles and are situated deeply in the substance of the brain. They are not common, nor are the other tumours which develop in the cerebral hemispheres, e.g. *colloid cyst* of the third ventricle, *papilloma* of the choroid plexus and *cholesteatoma*.

The pineal gland is situated in the posterior wall of the 3rd ventricle in the midline. A *pinealoma* is a tumour involving the pineal gland and may extend forwards to block the flow of C.S.F. so causing obstructive hydrocephalus (see Chapter 13). Other effects are variable, depending upon the main directions of growth. There may be compression or invasion of the cerebral hemispheres or the tumours may extend downwards compressing the posterior aspect of the mid-brain at the level of the corpora quadrigemina. This interferes with conjugate eye movements, typically causing defective upward gaze.

Pinealomas as a rule are not accessible for neurosurgical removal, but radiotherapy is effective in some. The hydrocephalus can be treated surgically, by making a shunt so that the C.S.F. can by-pass the obstruction and be absorbed. The most popular procedure now is to insert a Spitz-Holter valve; this is connected with a tube put into the lateral ventricle and a pumping device takes the C.S.F. into the jugular vein in the neck.

Pituitary tumours

The pituitary gland (often called the conductor of the endocrine orchestra because it secretes hormones which govern the other ductless glands) is situated at the base of the brain. Several types of tumour, depending on the main type of cell, may develop. The commonest are pituitary *adenomas* which are most frequently chromophobe, but eosinophil and basophil types also occur. *Craniopharyngioma* (i.e. tumours developing from embryonic remnants near the pituitary) are less common.

The main clinical effects of pituitary tumours are:

1. *Endocrine*

(a) Hypopituitarism—due to compression of the pituitary gland by the tumour interfering with production of one or more pituitary hormones, so causing secondary defects of gonadal (sex), adrenal or thyroid functions.

(b) Acromegaly—due to excessive production of growth hormone by the tumour cells.

(c) Cushing's syndrome—due to excessive production of adreno-corticotrophic hormone (A.C.T.H.) by the tumour cells.

2. *Compression of optic pathways*

The optic chiasm lies anterior to and above the pituitary fossa and is

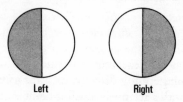

Left   Right

FIGURE 7. Bitemporal hemianopia

particularly vulnerable to pressure from an expanding pituitary tumour. The characteristic visual field defect which results from chiasmal compression is bitemporal hemianopia (see Fig. 7) due to damage to the nasal crossing fibres of the optic nerve which convey images from the temporal halves of both visual fields. Neurosurgical treatment is indicated for relief of failing vision.

3. The effects of suprasellar extension

Pituitary tumours can grow upwards out of the sella turcica and extend into the anterior or middle cranial fossae. This will compress the adjacent temporal or frontal areas of the cerebral hemispheres, causing focal epilepsy (e.g. with temporal lobe features) or motor deficits (e.g. facial weakness of U.M.N. type). Dysphasia is a rare complication as the speech area lies on the lateral surface of the dominant cerebral hemisphere.

CEREBELLAR TUMOURS

The main *primary* cerebellar tumours are:

(1) astrocytoma
(2) haemangioblastoma
(3) medulloblastoma

Astrocytoma of the cerebellum

In children astrocytomas occur more frequently in the cerebellum than in the cerebral hemispheres. They are often cystic, slowly progressive and invade the cerebellum and brain stem. Occasionally they originate in and remain confined to the brain stem.

Haemangioblastoma

These are usually benign encapsulated tumours, composed mainly of blood-vessel forming cells. Often cystic, they may contain large amounts of fluid with a relatively small tumour embedded in the wall (mural nodule). These tumours can often be removed completely.

Medulloblastoma

These occur almost invariably in children and are very malignant
tumours of the brain stem and cerebellar vermis. They are locally
invasive and extend deeply into the floor of the fourth ventricle.
Being friable, fragments break off and circulate in the C.S.F., becoming
attached to the surface of other parts of the neuraxis, e.g. the spinal
cord. This type of spread is called 'seeding'. Medulloblastomas are
initially radiosensitive but nearly always recur so that the prognosis
is poor.

METASTASES

Secondary tumours (metastases) in the cerebellum are not infrequent,
the commonest site of the primary tumour being the lung or breast.

ACOUSTIC NEUROMA

A neuroma or neurofibroma is a benign primary tumour which may
grow from the sheath of any (cranial or spinal) nerve. The commonest
cranial nerve to be affected is the 8th cranial (acoustic) nerve. Very
rarely there may be bilateral acoustic neuromas. In a small percentage
of cases (10–15%) an acoustic neuroma may be associated with multiple
neurofibromatosis (Von Recklinghausen's disease). In this condition,
the tumours grow on the peripheral nerves in the skin and subcutaneous
tissue; it is often associated with pigmented (café-au-lait) patches on
the skin. Skeletal deformities can develop and tumours on the spinal
nerve roots may compress the spinal cord.

An acoustic neuroma interferes with 8th nerve functions (auditory
and vestibular) causing unilateral deafness, tinnitus and vertigo. The
deafness is perceptive in type and progressive. Tinnitus is the hallucination of sound and the patient may be aware, for example, of a continuous hum or hiss in the affected ear. Vertigo is the hallucination of
movement, usually rotatory, similar to the sensation experienced
immediately after getting off a roundabout.

Situated in the cerebello-pontine angle, an acoustic neuroma will
also cause the following:

(1) involvement of other cranial nerves, particularly the 7th and

5th, resulting in facial weakness and numbness, including loss of the corneal reflex,

(2) compression of the cerebellar hemisphere with incoordination of the arm and leg on the same side, nystagmus and dysarthria,

(3) compression of the brain stem producing pyramidal (U.M.N.) signs,

(4) raised intracranial pressure—viz. headache, vomiting and papilloedema.

As the tumour is benign and encapsulated, removal is usually possible but owing to its situation there may be technical difficulties. Since an expanding tumour will eventually prove fatal from increase in intracranial pressure or compression of the brain stem, neurosurgery is advisable and, when the tumour is small, results are satisfactory. Unfortunately the 7th cranial nerve, being in such close proximity to the 8th nerve during its course from the brain stem to the facial canal, is frequently compressed by the tumour and may have to be sacrificed during removal of the tumour. The facial palsy which ensues is disfiguring and initially may cause dysarthria; patients usually learn to compensate for this and pronounce words quite clearly by talking out of the unaffected side of the mouth. Plastic surgery can improve the cosmetic effect and facio-hypoglossal nerve anastomosis provides reasonable function in the facial muscles, the unilateral paralysis and wasting of the tongue (resulting from division of the hypoglossal nerve) being relatively unimportant.

The dysarthria resulting from damage to the cerebellum or the lower cranial nerves often persists post-operatively and speech therapy is indicated to improve articulation. With involvement of the 10th cranial (vagus) nerve, nasal voice and dysphonia may occur but usually improve post-operatively.

CHAPTER 17
VASCULAR DISORDERS

Blood supply of the brain

Four arteries in the neck carry the blood supply to the brain, namely the internal carotid and vertebral arteries on each side. The internal carotid arteries pass through the foramen lacerum at the base of the skull to follow a tortuous intracranial course (the carotid syphon). Above this each gives off the ophthalmic artery and then terminates

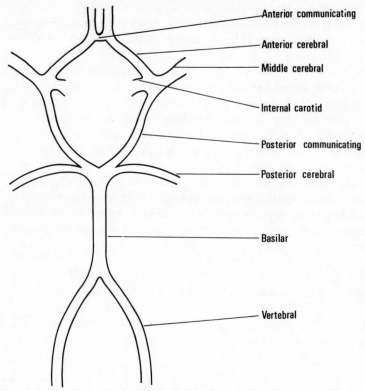

FIGURE 8. Diagram of the Circle of Willis. (From *The Management of Cerebro-vascular Disease*, by J. Marshall, 2nd ed. Churchill, London, 1968.)

by dividing into anterior and middle cerebral arteries. The vertebral arteries pass up through the vertebral canals in the transverse processes of the cervical vertebrae, coil around the arch of the atlas on each side and pass through the foramen magnum, above which they join to form the basilar artery; this artery ascends in the midline along the anterior aspect of the brain stem to which it gives off paired branches. At the upper level of the mid-brain the basilar artery terminates by dividing into the two posterior cerebral arteries. *The Circle of Willis* (see Fig. 8) is completed by the posterior communicating arteries, which join the posterior cerebral to the internal carotid arteries and by the anterior communicating artery which joins the right and left anterior cerebral arteries.

STROKES

A stroke is a catastrophic or potentially serious disorder of brain function due to interference with the circulation. The three main causes are:

1. haemorrhage
2. infarction
3. transient ischaemic attacks ('little strokes')

1. HAEMORRHAGE

Haemorrhage results from rupture of the wall of a blood vessel so that blood escapes from the circulation, either into the subarachnoid space (subarachnoid haemorrhage), the substance of the brain (intra-cerebral or intracerebellar) or into the ventricle (intraventricular); the blood may clot forming a haematoma.

Intracranial haemorrhage usually causes sudden headache, often with loss of consciousness. Within a few minutes, there are usually signs of meningeal irritation due to blood in the subarachnoid space, e.g. photophobia (dislike of light) and neck stiffness, which disappear if coma supervenes.

The commonest causes of intracranial haemorrhage are:

(1) atheroma and arteriosclerosis, with hypertension
(2) aneurysm and angioma
(3) bleeding diseases
(4) trauma

Atheroma and Arteriosclerosis

The three layers of a vessel wall are (1) the *intima* which is the inner endothelial lining, (2) the *media* or muscular and elastic layer, and (3) the *adventitia* which is the connective tissue surrounding the blood vessel. Atheroma is the name given to the change in the arteries due to deposition of plaques of cholesterol in the intima. It usually affects the smaller and medium sized arteries and causes narrowing of the lumen. Arteriosclerosis occurs when the elastic tissue degenerates, the wall of the artery becomes thickened, irregular and tortuous, and micro-aneurysms may form on the capillaries. High blood pressure (which is commonly associated with degenerative arterial disease) will further aggravate the liability of the vessel wall to rupture, resulting in haemorrhage.

Aneurysm

This is a dilation of the artery, usually at a point of bifurcation, due to congenital weakness in the media. Most aneurysms are found on the main arteries of the circle of Willis, approximately 30% arising from the anterior group (i.e. the anterior cerebral and anterior communicating arteries), 30% directly from the internal carotid artery, usually at the level of the junction with the posterior communicating artery and 30% from the middle cerebral arteries. The remaining 10% are situated on the various other intracranial arteries, i.e. vertebral and basilar or their branches, or on the peripheral branches of the cerebral arteries.

The wall of an aneurysm is more liable to rupture as the patient gets older, when atheromatous changes become superimposed and hypertension develops. The seriousness of rupture of an intracranial aneurysm is evidenced by the fact that about 50% of patients die within four weeks and few survive more than 2 or 3 haemorrhages.

Another complication occurs if the sac of the aneurysm enlarges and compresses the neighbouring structures; for example, compression of the third cranial (oculo-motor) nerve by an aneurysm of the internal carotid artery at its junction with the posterior communicating artery causes an oculo-motor palsy, viz. ptosis, dilated pupil and paralysis of the external ocular muscles (excluding the superior oblique and lateral rectus muscles).

Angioma

An angioma is a congenital malformation consisting of a mass of abnormal blood vessels. It may be situated within the substance of one cerebral hemisphere or the brain stem, or superficially on the surface, sometimes extending deeply into the cerebral hemisphere in the shape of a wedge. The size varies from minute angiomas visible only with a microscope to extremely large ones involving almost the whole of one hemisphere; they are supplied by some or all of the main arteries of the circle of Willis. Instead of blood taking its normal time and course through the capillaries of the brain, these congenital anomalies form large arterio-venous communications or shunts which tend to deprive the underlying area of the brain of its normal blood supply. The vessels making up the angioma are abnormally thin and liable to rupture so that subarachnoid or intracerebral haemorrhages are common complications. Rupture of an angioma tends to occur at an earlier age than with an aneurysm and is less commonly fatal so that there may be a history of several haemorrhages.

Other complications of angioma are epilepsy and persistent neurological deficits such as dysphasia, depending on which part of the brain is involved.

Bleeding diseases

Subarachnoid and intracerebral haemorrhages, often minute but multiple, can result from haemorrhagic diseases in which there is some general disorder of the clotting mechanism of the blood, e.g. when there is a deficiency of platelets as in thrombocytopenia and some cases of leukaemia. Intracranial haemorrhage may also occur as a complication of anticoagulant therapy.

Trauma

Head injuries may cause haemorrhage or contusion in the substance of the brain, sometimes with bleeding into the subarachnoid space (traumatic subarachnoid haemorrhage). Bleeding may also occur into the extradural or subdural spaces forming localised clots (extradural or subdural haematoma); the resultant rise in intracranial pressure can cause severe, even fatal, complications because of compression and distortion of the cerebral hemispheres or brain stem. In any severe head injury with intracranial haemorrhage there may be a fracture of the skull and concussion. Concussion is the 'knock-out' of brain function that follows a head injury, i.e. the immediate loss of consciousness, confusion and amnesia that are reversible and not due to any *visible* brain damage which may or may not coexist (see Chapter 19).

Investigations

Lumbar puncture in subarachnoid haemorrhage reveals uniformly blood-stained C.S.F. instead of the normally clear and colourless fluid. If the specimen is centrifuged or allowed to stand, the supernatant fluid has a yellow tinge (*xanthochromia*).

X-rays of the skull may show a fracture, or displacement of the calcified pineal gland, for example, by an intracranial haematoma. (The pineal gland appears calcified in the skull X-rays of about 50% of normal people and should be in the midline.) Echoencephalography (using an ultrasonoscope) may also indicate shift of midline structures and scanning techniques using radioactive isotopes may demonstrate the position and size of lesions. Recently the E.M.I. scanner using an X-ray technique called computerised transverse axial tomography has been introduced and has proved capable of demonstrating intracranial haemorrhages and distinguishing them from other intracranial lesions. Prior to this the most important diagnostic test was arteriography, a radiological technique involving the injection of a radio-opaque fluid into either of the carotid or vertebral arteries in the neck. The radio-opaque fluid is carried with the circulating blood into the intracranial blood vessels which are then revealed by X-rays. An intracranial haematoma (extradural, subdural or intracerebral) is demonstrated by displacement of the blood vessels; for example, instead of the anterior cerebral artery lying almost in the midline, it may be displaced towards the opposite side; an aneurysm is shown as a small diverticulum on an artery; an angioma as a tangle of knotted vessels on the surface of, and perhaps extending deeply into, one cerebral hemisphere; atheroma and arteriosclerosis are revealed by narrowing, irregularity and tortuousity of the arteries.

Treatment

Intracranial haematoma can be removed surgically. If an aneurysm is found, the management depends on its exact situation since many are now accessible to surgery by ligation or clipping of the neck or base of the aneurysm close to its junction with the wall of the artery. This prevents any future rupture as the aneurysmal sac is excluded from the circulation. An alternative method is to wrap a piece of muscle or synthetic material around the fundus of the sac to strengthen the wall and prevent any recurrent rupture. Yet another method of treatment is to reduce the pressure in the arteries leading to the aneurysm by ligation of the common carotid artery in the neck. When the patient is hypertensive, the blood pressure can be effectively lowered by hypotensive drugs.

2. INFARCTION

Infarction is death of tissue (necrosis) due to impairment of the blood supply (ischaemia). If the cells of the nervous system (neurones) are deprived of their blood supply for more than a few minutes, they cannot survive and there will be an area of cerebral infarction. The extent of the infarct and the resultant neurological deficits will depend not only on which vessel is obstructed but also on the capacity of neighbouring arteries to supplement the deficient blood supply, i.e. develop a *collateral circulation*.

The two main causes of prolonged or severe ischaemia sufficient to produce infarction are (a) thrombosis and (b) embolism.

(a) Thrombosis

Intravascular clot formation (thrombosis) is commonly due to atheroma with slowing of the blood flow. The clot causing the obstruction may develop either in the intra- or extra-cranial parts of the carotid and vertebral arteries; this is liable to result in cerebral infarction particularly if the intracranial vessels are arteriosclerotic, which reduces the capacity to form a collateral circulation.

Investigations

The cerebro-spinal fluid is nearly always clear (i.e. not obviously blood-stained) and carotid arteriography may show the point of obstruction in the affected artery. At least 20% of strokes are due to occlusion of the extracranial part of the internal carotid artery in the neck just above the bifurcation of the common carotid artery.

Treatment

In some cases it may be possible to remove the thrombus surgically, if it is near the origin of the internal carotid artery in the neck and if the block is not complete. This may be justified if serious cerebral deficit has not already developed, but the long term results of such procedures are still uncertain.

Anticoagulant therapy is contra-indicated in acute cerebral infarction due to thrombosis because of the danger of bleeding into the infarcted brain tissue. Severe hypertension can be treated with hypotensive drugs but care must be taken not to reduce the blood pressure below a certain level as this may further impair the cerebral circulation and interfere with recovery.

(b) Embolism

An embolus is a fragment of clot or other substance, e.g. fat, air, aggregations of platelets, fibrin or cholesterol, which is carried in the circulation from one part of the body and obstructs a blood vessel elsewhere. Embolism is liable to occur in various heart diseases, for example when the auricles are not contracting properly (auricular fibrillation) so that the blood in the auricles becomes stagnant and forms clots. Fragments break off, pass through the auricular-ventricular valves (mitral or tricuspid) to be expelled via the main arteries and carried in the circulation, eventually obstructing smaller blood vessels such as the cerebral arteries supplying the brain. If the obstruction is not relieved (for example by further fragmentation or absorption of the embolus) and if the collateral circulation is inadequate, the area of brain involved will become infarcted. Embolism also occurs in myo-cardial disease secondary to coronary thrombosis, i.e. a clot in the coronary arteries supplying the heart, so that there is infarction of the heart muscle (myocardial infarction). This may involve the inner lining of the heart (endocardium) with formation of a clot on the endocardial surface. If this fragments, emboli may then be carried via the aorta into any of the main arteries in the body and cerebral embolism may result.

Cerebral embolism presents with an extremely sudden disturbance of function, the resulting signs depending upon which part of the brain is rendered ischaemic. Dysphasia and hemiplegia due to a cerebral embolus will have an acute onset followed by improvement. Although recovery in some cases is slow and incomplete, in others there is no loss of consciousness and the prognosis is excellent. Specific medical or surgical treatment is directed to the underlying cause of the clot formation and anticoagulant therapy is used in some cases.

3. TRANSIENT ISCHAEMIC ATTACKS

Occlusion of blood vessels by thrombosis or embolism is not necessarily complete and the ischaemia may be insufficient to cause infarction. Transient ischaemic attacks (T.I.A.s) are temporary or relatively minor short-lived disturbances of cerebral function, sometimes referred to as 'little strokes'. Repeated T.I.A.s may be due to microembolism by atheromatous material and platelet-fibrin aggregates. A common site of origin of these microemboli is from an atheromatous plaque (patch of atheroma) on the internal carotid artery just above the bifurcation of the common carotid artery in the neck. T.I.A.s affecting the cerebral hemispheres, retina or brain stem are commonly encountered in arteriosclerotic patients with narrowing (stenosis) of the internal carotid or vertebral arteries. If this can be confirmed by arteriography and if the narrowed segment is localised in an accessible situation in a relatively young patient, it may be treated surgically. Carotid endarterectomy or reconstruction is highly successful in preventing both recurrent attacks and subsequent major strokes. Anticoagulant therapy may also be effective in some cases.

The vertebral arteries are vulnerable to obstruction in the vertebral canal of the cervical spine and in their upper part as they curve round the transverse processes of the atlas. Excessive or prolonged movements of the head and neck can interfere with the circulation via the vertebral arteries, particularly when these are arteriosclerotic. In middle aged and elderly subjects, there is often cervical spondylosis, i.e. degeneration of the cervical spine with narrowing of the disc spaces, the small joints becoming deformed with bony irregularities (osteophytes). These may impinge on the vertebral arteries and impede the circulation especially when the head is turned or the neck extended.

Transient ischaemic attacks affecting the brain stem are referred to as 'vertebro-basilar insufficiency'. The symptoms are due to the disturbances of brain stem function resulting from involvement of cranial nerve nuclei, e.g. defects of eye movements and diplopia (3rd, 4th and 6th), sensory loss on the face (5th), facial weakness (7th), tinnitus, deafness, vertigo and nystagmus (8th), loss of palatal sensation (9th), palatal weakness, dysphagia, dysphonia and dysarthria (10th, 11th and 12th). Involvement of the sympathetic fibres in the brain stem will cause Horner's syndrome (partial ptosis, constriction of the pupil, enophthalmos and loss of sweating on the forehead of the affected side). In addition there may be inco-ordination and ataxia of the limbs, nystagmus and ataxic dysarthria from ischaemia of the cerebellum and its connections.

As mentioned previously, if the ischaemia is prolonged beyond the critical period, infarction will result and the same neurological deficits may become permanent. Transient ischaemic episodes recurring repeatedly may thus herald the onset of a major stroke. Sometimes it is possible to relieve these transient attacks, for example by restriction of neck movements (using a collar).

Conditions causing fall in cardiac output and blood pressure also produce transient cerebral ischaemia and this is the mechanism of fainting (*syncope*). The fall in blood pressure results in defective blood supply to the brain stem and cerebral hemispheres producing the symptoms of faintness, dizziness, blurred vision and nausea etc. leading to loss of consciousness; the patient falls to the ground and this lowering of the head restores the blood supply to the brain so that recovery is rapid. There are many causes of syncope, e.g. vaso-vagal attacks, cough syncope, hypotension and cardiac disorders such as heart block (*Stokes-Adams attacks*). Sometimes it is necessary to monitor the electrocardiogram to demonstrate that T.I.A.s are related to a cardiac dysrhythmia.

Spasm of cerebral blood vessels (narrowing due to contraction of the muscle wall) is occasionally seen in arteriograms and at operation following subarachnoid haemorrhage. If the period of ischaemia is short, infarction does not occur and recovery follows when the spasm clears and the blood supply is restored. Spasm or vasoconstriction producing cerebral, retinal or brain stem ischaemia is also thought to account for the transient premonitory symptoms (e.g. visual, sensory and sometimes speech disturbances etc.) which occur in *migraine*, the headache being associated with the subsequent vasodilatation.

CHAPTER 18

INFECTIONS

Infections are the result of invasion of the body by micro-organisms such as bacteria and viruses. These organisms vary in virulence, i.e. their capacity to spread and cause disease.

The factors which determine the result of an infection are the resistance or susceptibility of the host tissues (a high standard of general health and well-being will tend to improve resistance to infection), the virulence of the infecting organism and the sensitivity of the organism to treatment.

Bacteria are microscopic organisms which are universally disseminated. Each organism consists of one cell which has the capacity to multiply but only some produce disease (i.e. are pathogenic). Bacteria have various shapes, e.g. round (cocci), rod shaped (bacilli), but a high-power microscope is necessary to see these.

Viruses are also unicellular organisms but are smaller than bacteria. Infections due to viruses include the common cold, influenza, measles, poliomyelitis, small pox and chicken pox, herpes simplex and zoster. Viruses may infect the nervous system and cause meningitis or encephalitis (inflammation of the meninges or brain). Encephalitis may be diffuse and involve large areas of the brain, or be localised and result in abscess formation. The herpes simplex virus causes a very severe form of encephalitis, the maximum inflammation frequently involving the temporal lobes.

Inflammation

Tissues which become infected with an organism produce an inflammatory reaction, i.e. there is redness and swelling due to increase of the local blood supply (vasodilatation) with seepage of fluid and white blood cells (leucocytes and macrophages). Necrosis in the centre of the inflamed area may lead to pus formation and a surrounding capsule is formed by fibrous tissue. The pus-filled cavity increases in size and at the point of least resistance comes to the surface, where it may burst spontaneously, or require surgical evacuation of the pus. Provided that the infection is overcome by virtue of the resistance of the tissues and treatment with appropriate antibiotics, the inflammatory reaction will subside.

Abscess

An abscess is a localised pocket of infection containing pus, e.g. a boil is an abscess in the skin. In some parts of the body, if the pus cannot be evacuated, the abscess increases in size and penetrates deeply to cause increasing damage by compression.

A cerebral abscess is the result of an infection which reaches the brain either by direct spread from the middle ear (otitis media), or sinuses (sinusitis), or via the blood stream e.g. from the lungs (pneumonia or pulmonary abscess). The cerebral abscess acts as an intracranial space-occupying lesion producing symptoms and signs of raised intracranial pressure, viz. headache, vomiting and papilloedema. Local effects are determined by its situation e.g. it may cause focal epilepsy or neurological signs, including dysphasia if the speech area is involved.

Otitis Media and Mastoiditis

Infection of the middle ear may penetrate the petrous bone spreading anteriorly into the middle cranial fossa to involve the temporal lobe, or posteriorly into the posterior fossa to involve the adjacent cerebellar hemisphere. Abscesses can form in other parts of the brain, even on the side opposite to the infected ear, and may be multiple, indicating that the spread has been via the blood stream.

Local meningeal reaction or rupture of an intracerebral abscess leads to meningitis. Other complications from otitis media include lateral sinus thrombosis and cortical thrombo-phlebitis.

The organisms that cause these infections are most commonly the staphylococcus, Bacterium coli, Haemophilus influenzae and Proteus.

Meningitis

Inflammation of the meninges usually results from spread of a local infection or is a complication of a systemic infection, frequently viral. Bacterial meningitis in adults may be due to the meningococcus or pneumococcus and in children to Haemophilus influenzae, although any of the bacteria already mentioned may be responsible. Meningo-coccal meningitis (cerebro-spinal or 'spotted fever') occurs in epidemic form and, before the discovery of sulphonamides and anbibiotics, was often fatal, but nowadays it is more amenable to treatment. It was called 'spotted-fever' because in fulminating cases, purpura (minute haemorrhagic spots) developed in the skin. Haemorrhage occasionally occurred in the adrenal glands causing death from adrenal failure.

Many of the complications of meningitis are the result of inflam-matory exudate forming mainly at the base of the brain, so damaging the cranial nerves. Involvement of the 8th cranial (auditory) nerves, causing deafness, is most frequent, but damage to this nerve can also result from the toxic effects of streptomycin (one of the antibiotics used in the treatment of tuberculosis).

Tuberculosis

Infection with the tubercle bacillus (T.B.) most commonly involves the lungs (pulmonary tuberculosis). All forms of tuberculosis including tuberculous meningitis are now relatively rare in England but still common in Asia. Tuberculous abscesses more often occur in the cerebellar than cerebral hemispheres and are complications of tuber-culosis of tissues elsewhere (e.g. the lungs), the infecting organisms (tubercle bacilli) being carried to the brain via the blood stream. As the tuberculous abscess enlarges, raised intracranial pressure develops. Alternatively a chronic granuloma (tuberculoma) is formed and may exist in the brain for months or even years without causing symptoms. It may become inactive and calcified showing up on plain X-rays of the skull as a rounded irregular calcified mass.

Syphilis

This is one of the venereal diseases which may produce local genital symptoms when contracted, and then remain latent to produce manifestations of involvement of the nervous system (neurosyphilis) many years later. There is also a congenital form of the disease due to transmission to the foetus by an infected mother. The spirochaete which causes syphilis, Treponema pallidum, is a cork-screw shaped micro-organism, which invades the tissues to cause the specific inflammatory reaction of the disease. Neurosyphilis is now relatively rare, but the classical types are still recognised.

General paralysis of the insane (G.P.I.)

G.P.I. develops after a latent period following the acute infection, sometimes as long as 10–20 years later. The disease affects the cerebral hemispheres causing generalised atrophy, particularly of the cortex. The mental, intellectual and personality deterioration (dementia) is progressive unless early treatment with penicillin is given. There are generalised tremors, involving particularly the hands, lips and tongue. The tremor of the hands is usually fine and rapid, but the tremor of the tongue is sometimes coarse with backwards and forwards movements, aptly described as 'trombone tremor'. Bilateral pyramidal signs with increased reflexes, clonus and extensor plantar responses are often present. There is a characteristic type of dysarthria which may be due to a combination of factors, viz. the tremor of the tongue, pseudobulbar palsy (due to bilateral upper motor neurone involvement), and cortical atrophy affecting the motor part of the speech area.

In all forms of neurosyphilis, pupillary abnormalities are frequently seen. The most characteristic is the *Argyll Robertson pupil*, which is small and irregular in outline; it does not react to light but does to accommodation. (Argyll Robertson was an Edinburgh ophthalmologist who first described these abnormalities.)

Tabes dorsalis

The clinical picture is due to involvement of the posterior horns of the spinal cord, the posterior root ganglia of the spinal nerves and the sensory components of the cranial nerves. The main effects of tabes, therefore, are on the sensory system, depending upon the distribution of the segments affected. Involvement of the posterior nerve roots and ganglia often results in severe pain which is typically shooting or lancinating in character (lightning pains) causing sudden horizontally or vertically directed stabs, usually affecting the legs. Various visceral crises with bouts of severe pain may involve, for example, the bladder, stomach or larynx.

Loss of sensation occurs in various parts of the body, particularly the legs, ulnar aspects of the forearms and hands, over the chest and on the face and nose. Loss of superficial pain sensation is tested with a pin and, instead of the pinprick, the patient feels only a blunt touch. There is loss of deep pain sensation which is tested by squeezing the muscles and tendons (e.g. the tendo-Achilles) which are normally pain-sensitive. Loss of temperature sensation results in inability to differentiate between hot and cold and patients may sustain burns without feeling pain. The sensory fibres conveying pain and temperature sensations cross to the opposite side of the spinal cord and ascend in the lateral spinothalamic tracts. The posterior roots also convey the senses of position and vibration, which are conveyed up the spinal cord by the fibres of the posterior columns. Because these are affected in patients with tabes dorsalis (the name literally means wasting of the dorsal columns), there is loss of position and vibration sense in the limbs. The position of various parts of the body can be checked visually, so the patient can compensate for loss of the sense of position, but there will be unsteadiness with a tendency to fall in the dark or with the eyes closed, e.g. when washing the face. Loss of position sense can be tested by asking the patient to stand up straight with the feet together; with the eyes open, balance is maintained but on closing the eyes, the patient sways and may fall due to loss of position sense in the feet and legs (Romberg's sign).

Because of interference with sensation to the skin, trophic changes may occur leading to ulceration which is often indolent and chronic. Interference with the sensation of joints leads to a painless form of arthropathy with gross deformities (Charcot's joints).

As a result of the loss of sensation from the bladder the patient may fail to appreciate when the bladder is full so that there is retention of urine, or overflow incontinence with an atonic bladder.

The loss of sensation also interferes with the reflex arc, so that the tendon reflexes in the limbs are reduced or absent.

Speech is not as a rule affected in tabes, except in cases having combined features of both tabes and G.P.I., which is then called *taboparesis*.

Meningo-vascular syphilis

As the name implies, the blood vessels and meninges are particularly involved. The meninges become inflamed and thickened due to a low grade meningitis in which headache is a marked feature. Thickening of the meninges at the base of the brain can also cause cranial nerve palsies. The lumen of the blood vessels, particularly those penetrating the meninges and supplying the surfaces of the brain, becomes narrowed and obliterated. Local areas of ischaemia result and cause focal epilepsy and neurological signs; according to the part involved, so aphasia,

monoplegia or hemiplegia, homonymous hemianopia or hemianaesthesia may develop.

Gumma

This is a mass of granulomatous tissue due to syphilis and can occur
in almost any part of the body, including the brain. An intracerebral
gumma is exceedingly rare but acts as a space-occupying lesion causing
raised intracranial pressure with focal neurological deficits depending
upon its situation.

The *differential diagnosis* of neurosyphilis includes many disorders of
the nervous system which it can resemble. Fortunately laboratory tests
of the serum and C.S.F. are of great diagnostic value. Of these, the
Wassermann Reaction (W.R.) is widely used, and is positive both in
the serum and C.S.F. in most patients with active neurosyphilis. More
refined tests have now been developed, including the treponemal
immobilisation (T.P.I.) and fluorescent treponemal absorption (F.T.A.)
tests. In some cases the W.R. becomes negative after treatment with
penicillin, but the T.P.I. and F.T.A. usually remain positive and so
give additional evidence of previous spirochaetal infection.

All forms of neurosyphilis are now rare, as the acute venereal
infection can be effectively treated with penicillin and other antibiotics. Penicillin is the best prophylactic and curative treatment of
neurosyphilis, and previous methods using malaria, arsenic and bismuth
preparations have been superseded.

Poliomyelitis

This is an infection of the anterior horn cells of the spinal cord and
motor nuclei of the cranial nerves in the brain stem by the poliomyelitis
virus. The acute stage lasts a few days with symptoms of a systemic
illness, meningitis and sometimes encephalitis. If enough anterior horn
cells in the spinal cord are involved paralysis of lower motor neurone
type occurs, typically in a patchy distribution and, if the motor nuclei
in the brain stem are affected, bulbar palsy occurs with dysarthria,
dysphonia and dysphagia (see Chapter 10).

Bulbar palsy and respiratory paralysis may necessitate artificial
respiration, either with a tank type of respirator or tracheostomy with
a pump respirator (intermittent positive pressure respirator—I.P.P.R.).

Not all cases develop paralysis but, in those that do, recovery can take place provided that sufficient anterior horn cells or motor nuclei remain undamaged. Dead neurones cannot be replaced but probably more than half the number of functioning cells have to be damaged before any clinical weakness results. After the acute stage of the illness, further recovery of function is possible because certain muscles are capable of retraining and hypertrophy to compensate for those affected.

The serious epidemics that used to occur can be prevented by vaccination so that acute poliomyelitis is now a rarity.

CHAPTER 19

TRAUMA

The type of speech disturbance resulting from head injury depends on the site and extent of the structural damage to the brain. Damage to the language area in the dominant cerebral hemisphere causes dysphasia, and damage to the brain stem or cerebellar connections causes dysarthria. Many head injuries are relatively minor and superficial and cause no obvious damage to the brain; even with a linear fracture of the vault of the skull, the brain may escape detectable damage. However, brain damage often occurs when there has been a fracture of the skull, particularly if bone fragments are depressed.

A violent blow or blunt injury delivered to the head, or the head hitting forcibly on a fixed surface, may or may not cut the scalp or fracture the skull, but the sudden acceleration or deceleration of the brain within the skull causes diffuse damage or extensive areas of focal damage determined by the force of the impact and by the shearing strains within the brain substance. If the injury causes a depressed fracture of the skull, the underlying cerebral cortex will suffer maximum damage, but there may also be 'contrecoup' or other more widespread effects.

With penetrating injuries (for example, a high-velocity bullet) there is penetration of the dura mater with direct damage to the brain which may be localised or extensive; the neurological signs reflect the site, depth and extent of the brain damage. Depression of the inner table of the skull may have to be elevated surgically, and fragments of bone driven into the brain together with the penetrating missile itself may have to be removed.

Diffuse damage in its mildest form is reflected by *concussion*, i.e. 'the knockout' of brain function as evidenced by loss of consciousness, confusion and amnesia following immediately on the head injury and due to brain damage which is not macroscopically visible. With severe injuries, in adition to concussion, there may also be shearing strains and tearing of nerve fibres as well as haemorrhages contributing to the disruption.

Head injuries do not necessarily cause concussion, so there may be

FIGURE 9. Appearance of brain at post-mortem. From *Traumatic Aphasia*, by W. Ritchie Russell and M.L.E. Espir, Oxford University Press, London, 1961.)

no loss of awareness or loss of memory, but if there is brain damage from a closed (non-penetrating) head injury, the patient is usually unconscious for at least a short time. On regaining consciousness, there may be a further period of confusion or disorientation, and after recovery the patient does not remember events during part or all of this period from the moment of impact. This is *post-traumatic amnesia* and, as it may continue after consciousness appears to have been regained, calculation of its duration should include the total period of unconsciousness and/or amnesia from the moment of impact until continuous memory is restored.

After recovery from concussion it is often evident that there has also been loss of memory for a period of time leading up to and immediately preceding the impact; this is known as *retrograde amnesia*. The duration of unconsciousness following a head injury and of the post-traumatic amnesia are largely dependent on and related to the severity of the head injury and brain damage.

Damage to the language (speech) area of the dominant cerebral hemisphere may be due to contusion or haemorrhage from closed head injury, compression from a depressed fracture or direct trauma from a penetrating wound.

A severe closed head injury usually causes generalised effects with concussion and the associated shearing strains may damage the brain stem. On the other hand a penetrating wound causes direct focal damage, and although there is often some concussion as well, this may be minimal so that focal damage is occasionally sustained with no loss of awareness nor amnesia.

An example of this was a soldier who sustained a wound of the Rolandic region in November 1944 causing transient motor aphasia, weakness of the right side of the face and numbness of the right arm; he remembered the wound and remained fully conscious. His legs were not affected and after being wounded he walked two miles to meet the stretcher bearers. Bone fragments and damaged brain were removed at operation and he made a good recovery. Some years later he was killed in an accident and figure 9 showed the position of the brain wound.

If damage is confined to the speech area, dysphasia may be the only deficit; other focal signs may also occur in isolation or in combination, according to the site and extent of damage.

Missile wounds may cause extensive damage, either due to indriven fragments of bone or haemorrhage. These may be fatal but, if not, the wound may be complicated by infection and abscess formation. Neurosurgical treatment is required to remove debris, pus, blood clots, bone fragments and the penetrating missile if accessible. 'Post-traumatic' epilepsy is liable to develop in approximately 50% of such cases; this risk is very small in cases of closed head injury, especially when there is not a depressed fracture nor intracranial haematoma, and when the post-traumatic amnesia is relatively short (i.e. less than 24 hours).

Widespread brain damage usually causes prolonged coma. Eventual recovery of consciousness may then be accompanied by dementia sometimes with severe motor, sensory or visual deficits. Maximum recovery usually occurs during the first $1\frac{1}{2}$–2 years after the injury, but disability—including dysphasia—is permanent in some cases. Speech therapy is indicated for dysphasia as soon as the patient can co-operate after the acute effects of the head injury, and should continue so long as progress is being made.

Diffuse bilateral cerebral damage may cause dysarthria as part of a pseudobulbar palsy. In other cases dysarthria results from damage to the brain stem or cerebellum due to torsion with tearing of nerve fibres and haemorrhages.

Fractures of the base of the skull can cause tearing of the arachnoid mater, with leakage of cerebro-spinal fluid (C.S.F.) via the nose or ear (C.S.F. rhinorrhoea and otorrhoea respectively). The tear can allow entry of pathogenic organisms with infection leading to meningitis and sometimes intracranial abscess formation. Fractures of the base of the skull may also cause damage to one or more of the cranial nerves. The filaments of the olfactory nerves traversing the cribriform plate in the anterior fossa of the skull may be torn and anosmia (loss of the sense of smell) is not an uncommon complication of severe head injuries, and sometimes occurs in this way even when there is no fracture. Occasionally the optic nerves or chiasma are damaged, and fractures of the petrous temporal bone are particularly liable to damage the acoustic or facial nerves, causing deafness or facial palsy (of L.M.N. type) on the affected side. Damage to the vestibular mechanism, particularly the labyrinth, causes vertigo. During recovery this tends to be aggravated for some time by changes of posture, so-called *positional vertigo*. Although this usually subsides spontaneously, it is often troublesome for several months or more. This may be part of a *post-traumatic syndrome*, associated with impairment of speech, memory and other intellectual faculties, together with changes in personality, mood and behaviour such as disinhibition. These may persist after severe head injuries especially when there has been frontal and temporal lobe damage. Other cases develop a *traumatic neurosis* in which the predominant symptoms are persistent headache, depression, anxiety and irritability. These patients also complain of inability to concentrate, forgetfulness and lethargy, and they often fail to resume work, but there are usually no objective physical signs. This condition may be associated with organic deficits, but it is usually encountered in those who have sustained relatively trivial head injuries causing no, or only brief, concussion and particularly when litigation is pending.

Most of the severe closed head injuries in civilian personnel result from road traffic accidents, especially in motor cyclists and car drivers, whereas penetrating wounds are the result of military action.

In children brain damage may occur during birth, or later as the result of 'non-accidental injuries'—the so-called 'battered baby syndrome'.

Intracranial haemorrhage due to traumatic rupture of blood vessels constitutes one of the most serious and often fatal complications of a head injury. Single or multiple haemorrhages of varying sizes occur in the substance of the brain, forming an intracerebral or intra-cerebellar haematoma, or within part of the ventricular system, i.e. intraventricular haemorrhage.

Bleeding may also take place directly into the subarachnoid space, i.e. *traumatic subarachnoid haemorrhage*. The blood then becomes mixed with the C.S.F. which will be revealed if lumbar puncture is done. The clinical signs of subarachnoid haemorrhage are due to irritation of the meninges by the extravasated blood, so that there is meningism consisting of headache, neck stiffness and photophobia. In mild cases the bleeding stops spontaneously, the blood in the C.S.F. is absorbed and recovery ensues.

A head injury can also cause haemorrhage into the subdural space due to rupture of the veins draining into the venous sinuses and the resulting collection of blood becomes sealed off to form a *subdural haematoma*. In the acute stages this may be associated with severe cerebral damage and a high mortality rate. In some cases a subdural haematoma increases in size more slowly so that after a few weeks or months following the head injury there are signs of compression of the brain with raised intracranial pressure. The diagnosis is sometimes difficult, as the history of a preceding head injury is not always obtained, but prompt investigation and neurosurgical treatment usually results in recovery.

Head injuries, particularly with skull fracture, sometimes damage the meningeal vessels and cause bleeding into the extradural space. This *extradural haemorrhage* may be rapidly fatal, but the diagnosis should be suspected if the head injury is followed by deterioration in the level of consciousness and dilatation of one or both pupils. Occasionally this occurs after a period of recovery following the initial concussion so that there is a 'lucid interval' before coma again supervenes. An emergency operation to remove the extradural collection of blood and relieve the brain compression is then essential.

SELECTED BIBLIOGRAPHY

Chapter 1

BRAIN, W.R. (1965) *Speech disorders*. 2nd ed. London, Butterworths.
CRITCHLEY, M. (1975) *Silent language*. London, Butterworths.
DE CECCO, J.P. (1964) *The psychology of language, thought and instruction*. London, Holt, Rinehart and Winston.
LOCKE, S., CAPLAN, D. and KELLAR, L. (1973) *A study in neurolinguistics*. Springfield, Ill., Thomas.
MASON, S.E. (ed.) (1963) *Signs, signals and symbols*. London, Methuen.

Chapter 2

BOWSHER, D. (1975) *Introduction to the anatomy and physiology o, the nervous system*. 3rd ed. Oxford, Blackwell Scientific.
BREWER, C.V. (1961) *The organisation of the central nervous system*. London, Heinemann.
CARTERETTE, E.C. (ed.) (1966) *Speech, language and communication;* proceedings of the third conference on brain function, November 1963. Berkeley, University of California Press.
CHERRY, C. (1957) *On human communication*. London, Chapman and Hall.
LURIA, A.R. (1973) *The working brain; an introduction to neuropsychology*. Harmondsworth, Penguin Books.
MILLIKAN, C.H. and DARLEY, F.L. (eds.) (1967) *Conference on brain mechanisms underlying speech and language;* proceedings of a conference held at Princeton, N.J., 1965. New York, Grune and Stratton.
NATHAN, P. (1969) *The nervous system*. Harmondsworth, Penguin Books.
RUSSELL, W.R. (1959) *Brain, memory, learning*. Oxford, Clarendon Press.
RUSSELL, W.R. (1963) Some anatomical aspects of aphasia. *Lancet*, **1**, 1173–1177.

Chapter 3

BARBIZET, J. (1970) *Human memory and its pathology*. San Francisco, Freeman.
KORSAKOFF (1887) *Vestnik Klin: sudebnoi psickiat- nevropatol*. St. Petersburg (Russian text).
NIELSEN, J.M. (1958) *Memory and amnesia*. Los Angeles, San Lucas Press.
PAPEZ, J.W. (1937) Proposed mechanism of emotion. *Arch. Neurol. Psychiat.* **38**, 725–743.
RIBOT, T.-A. (1882) *Diseases of memory*. New York, Appleton-Century-Crofts.
ROSE, F.C. (1973) Disorders of memory. *Brit. J. Hosp. Med.* **9**, 225–232.
ROSE, F.C. and SYMONDS, C.P. (1960) Persistent memory defect following encephalitis. *Brain* **83**, 195–212.

ROSE, S.P.R. (1968) Biochemical aspects of memory mechanisms. In: Davison, A.N. and Dobbing, J. (eds.) *Applied neurochemistry.* Oxford, Blackwell Scientific.

RUSSELL, W.R. (1971) *The traumatic amnesias.* London, Oxford University Press.

SYMONDS, C.P. (1966) Disorders of memory. *Brain* **89,** 625–644.

TALLAND, G.A. and WAUGH, N.C. (1969) *The pathology of memory.* London, Academic Press.

VICOTR, M., ADAMS, R.D. and COLLINS, G.H. (1971) *The Wernicke-Korsakoff Syndrome.* Philadelphia, F.A. Davis.

WHITTY, C.W.M. and ZANGWILL, O.L. (eds.) (1966) *Amnesia.* London, Butterworths.

Chapter 4

CRICHLEY, M. (1953) *The parietal lobes.* London, Arnold.

Chapter 5

BENTON, A.L. (ed.) (1969) *Contributions to clinical neuropsychology.* Chicago, Aldine Publishing Co.

BOUILLARD, J. (1865) Discussion sur la faculté du langage articulé. *Bull. Acad. Méd.* (Paris), **30,** 575.

GAZZANIGA, M. and HILLYARD, S.A. (1971) Language and speech capacity of the right hemisphere. *Neuropsychologia* **9,** 273–280.

HECAEN, H. and AJURIAGUERRA, J. de (1964) *Left handedness; manual superiority and cerebral dominance:* trans. from French. New York, Grune and Stratton.

MILNER, B., BRANCH, C. and RASMUSSEN, T. (1964) *Disorders of language, Ciba Foundation Symposium,* page 200 (ed. by de Reuck A.V.S. and O'Connor, M.). London, Churchill.

PENFIELD, W. and ROBERTS, L. (1959) *Speech and brain mechanisms.* Princeton, University Press.

ROSE, F.C. (1965) *8th International Congress of neurology;* proceedings. Amsterdam, Excerpta Medica.

RUSSELL, W.R. and Espir, M.L.E. (1961) *Traumatic aphasia.* London, Oxford University Press.

WYKE, M. (1971) Dysphasia: a review of recent progress. *British Medical Bulletin* **27,** no. 3, 211–217.

ZANGWILL, O.L. (1960) *Cerebral dominance and its relation to psychological function.* Edinburgh, Oliver and Boyd.

ZANGWILL, O.L. (1967) Speech and the minor hemisphere. *Acta Neurologica Belg.* **67,** 1013–1020.

Chapter 6

CRITCHLEY, M. (1970) *The dyslexic child.* 2nd ed. London, Heinemann Medical.

FLOW, R.M., GOFMAN, H.F. and LAWSON, L.I. (1965) *Reading disorders.* Philadelphia, F.A. Davis.

FRANKLIN, A.W. (ed.) (1962) *Word blindness or specific developmental dyslexia; proceedings of a conference on . . .* London, Pitman.

FRANKLIN, A.W. (ed.) (1965) *Children with communication problems; proceedings of a conference on* . . . London, Pitman.

HALLGREN, B. (1950) Specific dyslexia. *Acta Psych. Neurol.* suppl. **65**, 1–287.

INGRAM, T.T.S. (1969) Disorders of speech in childhood. *Brit. J. Hosp. Med.* **2**, 1608–1625.

RENFREW, C. and MURPHY, K. (eds.) (1964) *The child who does not talk.* London, Heinemann Medical for Spastics Society (Clinics in Developmental Medicine, no. 13).

WORSTER-DROUGHT, C. (1971) A usual form of acquired aphasia in children. *Developmental Medicine and Child Neurology* **13**, 563–571.

Chapter 7

WHETNALL, E. and FRY, D.B. (1964) *The deaf child.* London, Heinemann Medical.

The young deaf child; identification and management; proceedings of a conference held in Toronto, Canada 8–9 October, 1964. *Acta Oto-Laryngol.* suppl. 206.

Chapter 8

ANDREWS, G. and HARRIS, M. (1964) *The syndrome of stuttering.* London, Heinemann Medical for Spastics International (Clinics in Developmental Medicine, no. 17).

JOHNSON, W. (1961) *Stuttering.* Minneapolis, University of Minnesota Press.

JONES, R.K. (1966) Observations on stammering after localised cerebral injury. *J. Neurol. Neurosurg. Psychiat.* **29**, 192–195.

TIMMONS, B.A. and BOUDREAU, J.P. (1972) Auditory feedback as a major factor in stuttering. *J. Speech and Hearing Dis.* **37**, 476–484.

VAN RIPER, C. (1971) *The nature of stuttering.* Englewood Cliffs, N.J., Prentice-Hall.

WYKE, B. (1971) The neurology of stammering. *J. Psychosom. Research* **15**, 423–432.

ZANGWILL, O.L. (1960) *Cerebral dominance and its relation to psychological function.* Edinburgh, Oliver and Boyd.

Chapter 9

BENSON, D.F. and GESCHWIND, N. (1971) *The Aphasias and Related Disturbances.* In *Clinical Neurology*, Vol. 1 Chapter 8 (ed. by Baker, A.B. and Baker, L.H.). Hagerstown, Harper and Row.

BROCA, P.P. (1861) Perte de la parole: ramollissement chronique et destruction partielle du lobe antérieur gauche du cerveau. *Bull. Soc. Anthrop.* (Paris), **21**, 235.

BUTLER, R.B. and BENSON, D.F. (1974) Aphasia: a clinical-anatomical correlation. *Brit. J. Hosp. Med.* **12**, 211–217.

CRITCHLEY, M. (1970) *Aphasiology; and other aspects of language.* London, Arnold.

DARLEY, F.L. (1972) The efficacy of language rehabilitation in aphasia. *J. Speech and Hearing Dis.* **37**, 3–21.

DEJERINE, J.L. (1914) *Sémiologie des affections du système nerveux.* Paris, Masson et Cie.

GESCHWIND, N. (1971) Aphasia. *New England J. Med.* **284**, 654–656.
HEAD, H. (1926) *Aphasia and kindred disorders of speech.* 2 Vols. Cambridge, University Press.
HENSCHEN, S.E. (1920) Klinische und anatomische Beiträge zur Pathologie des Gehrins. Part 5, Über Aphasie, Amusie and Akalkulie. Part 6, Über sensorische Aphasie. Stockholm, Nordiska Bokhandeln.
HENSCHEN, S.E. (1922) Klinische und anatomische Beiträge zur Pathologie des Gehirns. Part 7, Über motorische Aphasie und Agraphie. Stockholm, Selbstverlag.
HOPKINS, A. (1975) The need for speech therapy for dysphasia following stroke, *Health Trends* **7**, 58–60.
JACKSON, J. HUGHLINGS (1932) *Selected writings* (ed. by Taylor, J.). London, Hodder and Stoughton.
JENKINS, J.J., JIMENEZ-PABON, E., SHAW, R.E. and SEFER JOYCE, W. (1970) *Schuell's Aphasia in Adults; Diagnosis, Prognosis and Treatment.* 2nd edn. Hagerstown. Harper and Row.
KERSCHENSTEINER, M., POECK, K. and BRUNNER, E. (1972) The fluency–non fluency dimension in the classification of aphasic speech. *Cortex* **8**, 233–247.
KLEIST, K. (1934) Kriegsverletzungen des Gehirns in ihrer Bedeutung für die Hirnlokalisation und Hirnpathologie. In Handbuch der Ärztlichen Erfahrungen im Weltkriege 1914/1918 (ed. by von Schjerning, O.). Vol. 4, Geistes-und Nervenkrankheiten (ed. by Bonhoeffer, K.), pp. 686–933. Leipzig, Barth.
MARIE, P. (1906) Revision de la question de l'aphasie; la troisième circonvolution frontale gauche ne joue aucun role spécial dans la fonction du langage. *Sem. med.* (Paris), **26**, 241.
MARIE, P. et FOIX, Ch. (1917) Les aphasies de guerre. *Revue Neurologique*, **24 (i)**, 53.
RIOCH, D.M. and WEINSTEIN, E.A. (1964) *Disorders of Communication.* Baltimore, Williams and Wilkins.
TROUSSEAU, A. (1964) De l'aphasie. *Gaz. Hop.* (Paris), **37**, 13.
WEPMAN, J.M. (1951) *Recovery from Aphasia.* New York, Ronald Press.
WEPMAN, J.M. (1973) Rehabilitation and the language disorders. In *Rehabilitation practices with the physically disabled* (ed. by Garnett, J.F. and Levine, E.S.). New York, Columbia University Press.
WILLIS, T. (1683) *Two Discourses concerning the Soul of Brutes.* London, Pordage.

Chapter 10

BICKERSTAFF, E.R. (1971) *Neurology for nurses.* 2nd ed. London, English Universities Press.

Chapter 11

WALTON, J.N. (1975) *Essentials of neurology.* 4th ed. London, Pitman.

Chapter 12

DRAPER, I.T. (1974) *Lecture notes on neurology.* 4th ed. Oxford, Blackwell Scientific.

Chapter 13

CARTER, C.O. (1962) *Human heredity*. Harmondsworth, Penguin Books.
LORING, J. (ed.) (1968) *Assessment of the cerebral palsied child for education*. London, Heinemann Medical for Spastics Society.
MECHAM, M.J., BERKO, M.J. and BERKO, F.G. (1960) *Speech therapy in cerebral palsy*. Springfield, Ill., Thomas.
ROBERTS, J.A.F. (1959) *An introduction to medical genetics*. 2nd ed. London, Oxford University Press.

Chapter 14

FAIRFIELD, L. (1954) *Epilepsy*. London, Duckworth.
SUTHERLAND, J.M., TAIT, H. and EADIE, M.J. (1974) *The epilepsies; modern diagnosis and treatment*. 2nd ed. Edinburgh, Churchill Livingstone.
AIRD, R.B. and WOODBURY, D.M. (1974) *The management of epilepsy*. Springfield, Ill., Thomas.

Chapter 15

BROMLEY, D.B. (1966) *The psychology of human ageing*. Harmondsworth, Penguin Books.
EYSENCK, H.J. (1962) *Know your own I.Q.* Harmondsworth, Penguin Books.
GATHERCOLE, C.E. (1968) *Assessment in clinical psychology*. Harmondsworth, Penguin Books.
TERWILLIGER, R.F. (1969) *Meaning and mind; study in the psychology of language*. London, Oxford University Press.

Chapter 16

OLIVER, L. (1969) *Removable intracranial tumours*. London, Heinemann Medical.

Chapter 17

MARSHALL, J. (1976) *The management of cerebro-vascular disease*. 3rd ed. Oxford, Blackwell Scientific.
MATTHEWS, W.B. (1975) *Practical neurology*. 3rd ed. Oxford, Blackwell Scientific.

Chapter 18

BRAIN, W.R. and WALTON, J. (1969) *Diseases of the nervous system*. 7th ed. London, Oxford University Press.

INDEX